The Nice Guys' Guide™ To Getting Girls

You CAN be a Nice Guy & STILL Attract Women!

by The Nice Guys' Institute™
featuring The Nice Guy™ (John Fate)
and The Nice Guys™

Edited by
Laura Nathan

Please e-mail us at:
TheNiceGuys@TheNiceGuysGuide.com

ajackal publishing
Chesapeake VA

Visit our website at www.TheNiceGuysGuide.com
Contact us at TheNiceGuys@TheNiceGuysGuide.com

Visit Ajackal Publishing website at www.ajackal.com

First printing 2004

ISBN   0-9746042-8-3

LCCN   2003096950

Library of Congress Cataloging-in-Publication Data
The Nice Guys' Guide™ To Getting Girls: You CAN be a Nice Guy & STILL Attract Women! / The Nice Guys' Institute™ featuring The Nice Guy™ (John Fate) and The Nice Guys™.
P.cm.
ISBN: 0974604283

CONTENTS

CONTENTS

To Oscar, the original Nice Guy

ACKNOWLEDGMENTS

Editor: *Laura Nathan*

Cover Design: *Joseph Williams*

Thanks to all of our families and friends, for all that you've taught us about relationships.

– The Nice Guy™
and The Nice Guys™

Other Products by The Nice Guys™:

Make Every Girl Want You™
by John Fate (The Nice Guy™), Steve Reil

The Nice Guys' Guide™ Audio Series

The Nice Guys' Guide to Getting Girls 2™

Please see www.TheNiceGuysGuide.com for
the latest from The Nice Guys' Institute™!

The Nice Guys™ have appeared on:

The O'Reilly Factor

The Other Half

MTV's Big Urban Myth Show

The Ricki Lake Show

Naked New York

Jamie (White) & Danny (Bonaduce) Show

Don & Mike

Bubba the Love Sponge

Bottom Line Radio

Elvis Duran & The Z Morning Zoo

The Morning Madhouse

FNX Morning Show

Paul & Young Ron

...and others, too numerous to name!

WARNING—DISCLAIMER

This book is designed to provide information on making yourself more attractive to women. It is sold with the understanding that the publisher and authors are not engaged in rendering counseling or other professional services. If expert assistance is required, the services of a competent professional should be sought.

It is not the purpose of this manual to offer all-inclusive information on this topic, but rather to start you off on a path toward forming great relationships with women. You are urged to read all the available material, learn as much as possible about the subject, and tailor the information to your individual needs.

The techniques in this book are not a scheme designed to get sex. Anyone who decides to implement these techniques must expect to invest a lot of time and patience into it. The techniques in this book are powerful, and many have used them with great success. As you implement these techniques, be sure to practice safe sex and use contraceptives.

Every effort has been made to make this manual as complete and as accurate as possible (although the names and specific details in many stories have been changed to protect our friends' privacy). However, there may be mistakes, both typographical and in content. Therefore, this text should be used only as a general guide and not as the ultimate authority on making yourself more attractive to women.

The purpose of this book is to educate and entertain. The authors and Ajackal Publishing shall have neither liability nor responsibility to any person or entity with respect to any loss or damage caused (including but not limited to emotional damage), or alleged to have been caused, directly or indirectly, by the information contained in this book.

If you do not wish to be bound by the preceding, you may return this book to the publisher for a full refund.

Chapter 1 – The Nice Guys' Guide™ to Being an Attractive Nice Guy

This book is intended to be a sequel to *Make Every Girl Want You™*, the book that I co-authored with my good friend Steve Reil. We wrote that book – and this one – not because we were natural-born ladies' men looking to teach some old dogs new tricks, but because we know firsthand what it's like to go for months or even years without a date. Back in college, there was a good chance that if you looked up the word "pathetic" in the dictionary, you would find the definition followed by, "See also: 'John Fate' and 'Steve Reil.'" In those days, Steve and I didn't just fail miserably at wooing women to sleep with us – much less date us! – but we couldn't get women to give us the time of day if our lives depended on it. It often felt as if every woman on earth had signed a pact and agreed not to acknowledge our very existence.

Oh, sure, if the girl sitting next to me in class didn't understand something, she might ask me for clarification. I might have even chatted with her briefly during class. But if I saw her at a bar or a frat party later that night, I would be lucky if I got more than a thirty-second conversation out of her. Truth be told, I was usually not even that lucky.

Why was I so pathetic? Because I was a "nice guy." Maybe you can relate to this. To this very day, I am still a nice guy. And that's about all I've got going for me. I'm not rich, I'm not famous, and I'm not particularly good-looking. One of the first things Steve and I recognized, when we started observing why we were so pathetic, is that there are three categories of guys who seem to get all of the women. Guys who are:

1. Rich,
2. Famous, or
3. Good-looking

Unfortunately, like 90% of the other guys in this world, I had none of these three things going for me. I was not rich, not famous, and not good-looking; I was merely an average, nice guy.

For a period of time during college, I was so desperate for a date that I decided to abandon my natural "nice guy" personality for a while. I thought that acting like a rich, famous, or good-looking guy might cause the women to finally flock to me – or at least give me the time of day – so I put on this cocky, arrogant attitude when approaching the sex that I desired. Since neither this book nor its precursor is entitled *The Jerk's Guide to Getting Girls*, you've probably guessed correctly that this plan backfired. Although I didn't think it was possible, women wanted to be around me even less when I acted like someone I wasn't! So the moral to the story is that if you're not rich, famous, or good-looking, don't try to pretend you are and expect to reap some sort of benefit. Nice guys like us need our own approach to women.

After we graduated from college, Steve and I were so fed up with our pathetic lives that we decided we had to take action. Thinking like the engineering majors that we were, we decided to take an analytical approach to studying women. So, we came up with a game plan: For the next few months, we would only try to befriend women. We wouldn't try to date them; we wouldn't try to sleep with them. We would simply make it a point to become friends with every woman we met.

We began implementing this plan, and within a few months, we had a few dozen female friends! We would go out to bars and parties with these women and observe other guys hitting on them. We learned what worked and what didn't. The best part was that since we were friends with these women, they would debrief us after guys hit on them. They would say things like:

"Ugh, I can't believe that guy wouldn't shut up about med school."

"Wow, that guy had the most beautiful eyes!"

"Ugh, did that guy seriously think I wanted to hear non-stop about his boat? Talk about self-absorbed!"

"Wow, I really enjoyed talking to that guy. I didn't even feel like he was hitting on me."

While constantly capitalizing on the expertise of our newfound female friends, Steve and I also began studying our friend Oscar. Oscar, the nicest guy you'll ever meet, was a completely average guy like us: not rich, not famous, and not exceptionally good-looking. Yet, somehow, Oscar was constantly surrounded by beautiful women. Oscar was always dating these women; he was always sleeping with these women. Oscar had a date whenever he wanted one. His success with women was an enigma to Steve and me, so we decided that we would also study Oscar to figure out what it was about this seemingly-average nice guy that made him so attractive to women.

Make Every Girl Want You™ was our first attempt to share everything we learned about women with guys. Because of the tremendous success of that book, I have since started The Nice Guys' Institute™, which seeks to help other "nice guys" make themselves more desirable to women without turning into jerks. In fact, I have written this book with the help of The Nice Guys™, a group of guys that I recruited to help other nice guys. I chose to write this book in first-person singular as if I am the only author because it reads more smoothly that way. However, in reality, this book is a compilation of both my own discoveries and things that I have learned from The Nice Guys™, so I want to thank The Nice Guys™ for all of their help.

In the pages that follow, we have attempted to answer the most common questions that we've received from you, the readers of *Make Every Girl Want You*™ and the attendees of our courses. First, a word of warning: Much of the material in this book is written with the assumption that you have read *Make Every Girl Want You*™. Many of the concepts as well as the terminology that Steve and I introduced in that book provide the basis for this follow-up book; therefore, I strongly advise you to at least peruse our first book before reading any further.

I have written this book in a very different style than *Make Every Girl Want You*™, however. That book is meant to be an overview of how to meet women. It walks you though step-by-step, one chapter at a time: where to meet women, how to approach them, how to strike up a conversation, how to get contact info (and *correct* contact info!), how to ask a woman out, how to plan the first few dates, all the way up to having a successful, fulfilling relationship.

This book, on the other hand, really isn't a step-by-step guide at all. Rather, this book is a series of short articles. With the release and subsequent success of *Make Every Girl Want You*™, I have received thousands of questions via e-mail, in the courses I have taught, and in interviews that I've conducted. During the course of receiving these questions, I realized that *Make Every Girl Want You*™ left many questions unanswered, so I have attempted to answer those questions in the pages that follow.

The tone of this book differs as well. Written in a stream of consciousness style, this book is comprised of a series of articles that address specific questions posed to me or things that have naturally occurred to me or The Nice Guys™ as we experience life. As with *Make Every Girl Want You*™, the advice in this book is based on everything we've learned from our observation of and conversations with two sources:

1. Our many female friends
2. Oscar

Oscar epitomizes what every guy wants to be – a truly nice guy whom women love. Nowadays, as the founder of The Nice Guys' Institute™, I am frequently referred to as The Nice Guy™. However, I always say that Oscar was the original Nice Guy since I can't imagine that there would've been a Nice Guys' Institute™ if Oscar hadn't inspired me.

Before we move on to the substance of the book, let me briefly answer a question that I hear every time that I teach a course:

"Why don't you just ask Oscar how he does it?!?"

I tried that, but unfortunately, it's not really something that he can explain. Oscar has never taken the time to ponder why so many women are attracted to him. He just behaves the way that was naturally engrained in him, which I'm sure was some magical combination of genetics and his upbringing, such that everything in him somehow aligned to create the perfect Nice Guy. If only we could all be so lucky. Since Oscar himself didn't even have the answer to our million-dollar question, all we could do was watch, observe, and take notes. Hopefully, you'll like what we've learned. So read on to find out how to be a Nice Guy and *still* be attractive to women!

But first, I'd like to close this chapter by presenting six of my favorite testimonials. Since the release of *Make Every Girl Want You*™, we have received thousands of testimonials, both from men and women, thanking us for our books and courses. I'd now like to present six of my favorite, to illustrate how our books and courses have helped others, and how they will help you too.

From Robert, a 34-year-old man who has been married for eight years:

> "Our marriage had reached the point where we'd only had sex 3 times in the last 5 years. I wasn't even sure if she still loved me anymore.
>
> I tried a million things, bringing her flowers, taking her out to nice dinners, buying her jewelry. Still nothing. I couldn't even get her to talk about what was wrong with our marriage. Then, a friend of mine got me your book on a whim. He said, 'Hey, Robert. Try reading this. It might help.' And it did, CCR has changed my life!
>
> Not only is our sex life improved, but I feel like, for the first time in about 5 or 6 years, my wife and I actually understand each other. And we enjoy spending time

together once again. Thanks John & Steve
for saving my marriage."

From Michael, a 19-year-old college student:

"I've never had much luck with girls. In
fact, as much as it hurts me to write this,
I made it to 19 as a virgin. Don't get me
wrong, I've been out on dates. But I guess
the problem is that I can never get to the
3rd date, if you know what I mean. I just
really had no clue how to behave on a
date. I read your book cover to cover, and
then went back and read it a 2nd time.

A week later, I was sitting next to this
really hot girl in my chemistry class. I
struck up a conversation, exactly as you
guys instructed. That weekend, I found
myself having sushi with her. Only this
date was different. It was unlike any date
I've ever been on. I could tell that she was
actually digging me! I don't think she
looked at her watch once the entire time.

Best thing is, I didn't even need a 3rd date,
because 3 nights later we went out again
and she had sex with me! Thank you.
Thank you. Thank you."

From Lisa, a single gal who withheld her age:

"I bought a copy for my friend, Harold.
Harold's a great guy. I've been friends with
him for 8 years, and let me just say that
he has not had much success with the
ladies. Which really isn't fair, because he's
the world's sweetest guy. Of course, as a
woman, I can kind of understand why he
doesn't have success with women. But the

thing is, as much as I've tried to explain it to him, he just doesn't get it.

So I heard you guys on a radio show, and decided to buy your book for him. You guys said in 150 pages what I haven't been able to get Harold to understand in 8 years! Harold just has so much more confidence now. I can tell when I'm around him that he actually, finally, feels comfortable interacting with women. Sure, he's not a walking, talking babe magnet, but he's so much better off.

In fact, I recently introduced him to a couple of my female friends, who have both since asked about him. I mean, *my* friends – asking about Harold? That just doesn't happen! I'm almost starting to get jealous! Thanks guys, for a great book. I think every girl should buy it for her platonic male friends!"

From Corey, a 25-year-old professional:

"It's been a few years since I graduated from college. I have a good job and live in the city now, but man it's so much tougher to meet women than it was in college. In college, there were girls over at the frat house all the time. It was so easy to hook-up. Now, I can't even figure out where to meet women, let alone hook-up.

I ordered your book, and read it cover to cover in an hour. I discovered that my main problem is that I was looking for girls in all of the wrong places. Great book, guys—thanks a ton. I've already told all of my friends about it."

From Roger, who is 37 years old and divorced:

> "I finally understand why my first marriage failed. And let me tell you, until now I was clueless. I read your guys' book, because I'm single now. And I really read it for tips on where to meet women. But what really helped me is that you pointed out every single thing I did wrong in my first marriage.
>
> I'm dating someone now, and I definitely want to get married again someday. I don't know if it'll be to her, but I feel like I finally know what it will take to make a marriage work. I would recommend your book to any guy who wants to make his second marriage work."

From Julia, who is married—happily now—and requested that we not print her age:

> "I've been trying for years to get Bill to read 'relationship books.' But I haven't been able to get him to read a damn one. I saw you guys on TV, and figured—what the hell—I'll get your book, basically as a last resort. I gave it to Bill, and he read the entire thing that night.
>
> Afterward, he came up to me, gave me a big hug, and said: 'Honey, I have 2 things to tell you. #1: I want you to know how beautiful you are. And #2: I'm sorry I haven't told you that in 13 years.'"

Part I The Nice Guys' Guide™ to Meeting Women

In the "Getting Started: How to Meet Women" chapter of Make Every Girl Want You™, Steve and I introduced the three types of environments in which to meet women: Naturally-Inviting, Moderately-Inviting, and Bothersome Environments. In Part I of The Nice Guys' Guide™, I will offer further advice on where to meet women and how to approach them in different types of environments that we at The Nice Guys' Institute™ have discovered since Steve and I wrote Make Every Girl Want You™.

Chapter 2 – The Nice Guys' Guide™ to the Best Types of Bars

In *Make Every Girl Want You™*, Steve and I discussed the challenges of meeting – and actually talking to – women in Bothersome Environments such as bars. We explained why these locales are such difficult places to approach women and the importance of knowing when to move on.

Yet, I often get asked what the best places for picking up women are. Most men assume that there's some holy grail for meeting beautiful women, some place that they haven't yet discovered where thousands of beautiful women venture and sit all day long, waiting for men like you and me to approach them. Unfortunately, such a place doesn't actually exist, but I can point you in the direction of these women by offering some advice on characteristics to look for when choosing a bar.

The next time you go out to try your luck with women, keep in mind that your success – or the lack thereof – isn't based on luck. Instead, consider the following guidelines your new secret to success:

1. Avoid bars with an open floor plan

For starters, bars with an open floor plan tend to be the single man's worst enemy. I feel really uncomfortable spotting a woman on the other side of the bar, making eye contact, and then having to walk what feels like nine miles across the room to talk to her. On some occasions, the woman is gone by the time I get there. Other times, some other guy has approached her in the interim.

In both cases, I inevitably miss out on what might have been good conversation, a date, or perhaps something more. While there are certainly other fish in the sea, there's no reason to continue falling into the trap of the open floor plan of missed opportunities. That's why my favorite bars are those that have a lot of tables really close together, making it easy – and convenient – for you to strike up a conversation with the women at the table right next to yours.

2. Look for bars with long, communal tables

Much like bars with many tables close together, bars with long, communal tables typically provide a great environment for meeting new people. For instance, I was at a small bar a few nights ago in the East Village in Manhattan. There weren't many tables, but the tables were probably eight to ten feet long. When I looked around, I noticed that there were two or three different groups sitting at each table. There was generally one group of people at each end of the table as well as a couple of people in the middle who didn't know either party.

This setup was great. I was able to walk up to a table where three good-looking women were sitting at the other end of the table. I hung out with my friends, and we chatted for a bit. After a little while, I struck up a conversation with the women at the other end of our table. Starting a conversation with them was easy since they were seated a mere three feet away from me.

3. Try your hand at lounges

If the term "lounge chair" is any indication of the comfortable environment provided by lounges, you can rest assured that these locales provide a relaxing atmosphere for meeting women. Taking full advantage of the fact that lounges typically have groups of chairs facing each other and couches scattered around the bar, I usually prefer to find some empty chairs or couch space where some beautiful women are already sitting when I enter the lounge. Using the same approach that I use with long, communal tables, I usually sit down and chat with whomever I'm with. Then, after a few minutes, I'll strike up a conversation with the women sitting near me. Thanks to the comfortable, laid-back atmosphere of a lounge, this really is as simple as it sounds. My friend Olivia had this to say about some guys she met in a lounge a few weeks ago:

> "I was sitting with some friends of mine, near the back, on this row of couches. This group of guys walked up. They didn't walk right up and start talking to us. But they did sit in the same group of couches back there, and were just hanging out by themselves. Finally, one of the guys turned around and joined our conversation. He wasn't rude or anything. I can't remember what we were talking about, but he was very friendly.
>
> He said something like, 'I'm sorry to interrupt, did I just hear you guys talking about...' And next thing you knew, we

were talking to the whole group of guys. It was fun – we gave them our e-mail addresses, and we've all hung out a couple of times since them!"

4. Meet women in the bathroom line

Another great way to meet women at bars is to frequent bars that have long bathroom lines out the door, where the men's and women's lines are right next to each other. Striking up a conversation with women in the bathroom line is extremely easy since women are standing around for a while with nothing to do.

I'm never so bold as to ask for a woman's contact info while standing in the bathroom line, but I'll certainly strike up a conversation and chat for a few minutes. That way I feel much more comfortable – and confident – approaching her later in the evening since I've already met her and can rehash something that we discussed during our earlier conversation in the bathroom line.

5. Meet women at the bar while ordering a drink

For the same reasons that I like bars with long bathroom lines, I prefer bars that have a really long bar area where a lot of people can gather and stand around while waiting for their drinks. Here, just like in the bathroom line, women often stand around waiting without anything to do. In these situations, women tend to appreciate you striking up casual conversations with them.

Sometimes, rather than making the long walk over to talk to a woman that I spot early in the evening, I'll wait until she goes to get a drink or use the restroom. I'll then casually saunter over and strike up a conversation.

When striking up a conversation at the bar, I follow the same approach as in the bathroom line. I rarely get a woman's contact information while standing at the bar, but I at least establish a connection so that when I go up to talk to her later in the evening, she welcomes me as someone she recognizes rather than treating me like a total stranger.

Every rule that I've listed so far in this chapter is based on my observation of Oscar. Oscar never walks across the room to approach a random woman. Why? Because he knows that that puts him in a very awkward, uncomfortable situation, and that's not what Oscar is about. What Oscar is great at, however, is striking up conversation with the person standing next to him. If he's interested in talking to a woman across the room, he waits until he's next to her, which he does by proactively grabbing the next table over or strategically positioning himself next to her at the bar or in the bathroom line.

It never fails. Whenever I'm out with Oscar and he gets up to go to the bathroom or goes to the bar to grab drinks, I always look up a minute or two later and see him chatting with the person standing next to him. It isn't always a beautiful woman. Hell, it isn't even always a woman. Sometimes he's just chatting with the guy standing next to him about sports or which bar serves the best buffalo wings.

Why does Oscar have such an easy time meeting new people – and women in particular? Let's just say that Oscar maintains a completely different attitude than every other guy when he goes out at night. When Oscar approaches women, he truly maintains this mindset:

> "She looks like a fun, interesting person. I'd like to chat with her."

When Oscar goes out at night, he doesn't think of it in terms of picking up women. As a matter of fact, if you see him talking to a woman and say something along the lines of, "Hey, Oscar – are you trying to pick up that blond girl?" he always responds with something like

"Nah, I wasn't trying to pick her up – I was just chatting with her. We had a great conversation about her trip to Europe." Sure, some people may talk like this, but Oscar really means it when he says he was "just chatting with her."

When I talk about Oscar, many people think that he has some magical quality that enables him to walk up to any woman anywhere and have her phone number – if not more – within a few short minutes. But Oscar doesn't have superhero powers or a magic wand. What sets Oscar apart from everyone else I know is simply his ability – and willingness – to strike up a conversation anywhere at any time with anyone – men and women alike. Because Oscar has a really friendly, laid-back personality and is never afraid to talk to anyone, he approaches women with ease.

After observing Oscar, I have changed my attitude. Now when I go out at night, or even when I'm in a bookstore or grocery store, I also maintain the mindset that I'm not trying to pick up women. I merely engage people in conversation. I'll talk to the guy next to me in the checkout line at the grocery store, and I'll talk to a beautiful woman sitting beside me in a deli.

As you can see from the guidelines so far in this chapter, this isn't rocket science. These aren't groundbreaking, revolutionary techniques for meeting women. They are merely small changes that you can make to put yourself in close proximity to good-looking women so that you can naturally strike up conversations with them just as Oscar has always done, and as I now do.

6. Don't interrupt women in conversation

While it certainly can pay to be chatty and willing to talk to anyone, there are times when you should be patient and hold your tongue if you want to succeed in meeting women. As my friend Cathleen informed me, the problem that most guys face when approaching

women in a bar is their tendency to interrupt women in
mid-conversation:

> "You know, when I go out to a bar, I don't
> mind talking with some guys. But what
> really bothers me – and all of my
> girlfriends for that matter – is when a guy
> or two approaches us when we're already
> engaged in conversation. This puts me in
> a very awkward position.
>
> It's not that I don't want to talk to the guy.
> But if I start talking to him, then I'm
> offending my friend by cutting her off in
> the middle of her story. It sends the
> message to my friend, 'I'd rather talk to
> this random guy than you.' I know I would
> be offended if one of my friends started
> talking to a random guy while she was in
> the middle of a conversation with me.
>
> It's a shame because I've had plenty of
> guys approach me – guys who I would
> gladly talk to – but they always seem to
> approach me at the wrong time, like when
> I'm in the middle of a conversation with
> one of my friends. So I have to brush the
> guy off.
>
> I wish there was a way to tell the guy,
> 'Talk to me at the bar later. I can't talk
> right now!' When I'm just standing around
> waiting for drinks at the bar, that's the
> best time to approach me. That's when I'm
> likely to want to talk. That's how I've met
> most guys at a bar.
>
> You'd think guys would know this basic
> 'pick-up etiquette,' but it's quite obvious
> that very few guys actually do."

7. Shoot pool or play darts

I've found that shooting pool or playing darts is a great way to meet women, assuming that there are women standing nearby. On multiple occasions, a friend and I have started shooting pool for the sole purpose of meeting women. If the pool table is isolated from the rest of the bar, this strategy will inevitably fail. However, if the pool table is located in close proximity to the action, then it's very natural to invite some women standing nearby to play a little two-on-two.

In one of my all-time favorite bars, the pool table is right next to the women's restroom, which always has a line. Women standing in line inevitably turn and watch whoever is shooting pool since there's not much else for them to do (unless, of course, there's a guy waiting in line to use the men's restroom to talk to!). Whenever you shoot from the end of the table nearest the restroom, you'll inevitably find yourself standing beside two or three women afterwards. It's very easy to turn to them and say something like, "Wow! I can't believe I missed such an easy shot," followed by, "Do you shoot pool?" Whenever a friend and I shoot pool at this particular bar, we always end up playing with some women we met in the bathroom line, and often times, leave with their contact info!

Chapter 3 – The Nice Guys' Guide™ to Airports, Gyms, and Cruises

In *Make Every Girl Want You*™, Steve and I divided the places where you can meet women into three categories: Naturally-Inviting Environments, Moderately-Inviting Environments, and Bothersome Environments. We explained what locations fit into each category, in which locales women *prefer* to meet guys, and the strategy for meeting women in each environment. In this chapter, I introduce three new places where you can meet women and explain how to do so.

This chapter is actually more like three separate articles that I wrote at three different times. I wrote the first section about meeting women at the airport while sitting in LaGuardia Airport. I wrote the next article about meeting women at the gym after being interviewed for an article for *Men's Health*. The final article about meeting women on a cruise was written while on board a cruise I took recently. Hopefully, my good fortune with women in these locales will inspire you to approach some women the next time you're at the airport, working out at the gym, or on a cruise. Who knows, you might even start going to the gym, the airport, or taking cruises simply to meet women!

Airports

I'm sitting here in the food court of the US Airways terminal at LaGuardia Airport. In addition to a handful of restaurants, I've noticed that there are a lot of beautiful women here, many of whom are sitting alone. Wow, I think I've found a new hotspot for meeting women – airports!

There is a drop-dead gorgeous woman sitting two seats down from me. She has long dark hair and beautiful brown eyes. She appears to be of Persian descent. Hold on one moment; I'm going to try to strike up a conversation with her . . .

OK, I'm back. I just spent the last twenty minutes chatting with Erica. She's an actress, went to NYU, and now lives in Brooklyn. And the greatest part about this is that she just happens to be on my flight to Norfolk! I've never even thought of an airport as a great place to meet women, but I have some advice for guys: Forget what the airlines say about getting to the airport two hours early; from now on, get there five hours before your flight! Now don't get me wrong; I'm not telling you to go to the airport just to pick up women. With today's security measures, you can't even get past security unless you have a ticket with today's date on it. However, if you happen to find yourself in an airport, I suggest that you make the most of it. With this in mind, let's discuss some general guidelines for meeting women at the airport.

1. Sit near a woman in the food court or a restaurant

It appears that the food court and restaurants at an airport are the best places to meet women. The food court here at LaGuardia seems to be particularly conducive to meeting women since the rows of long tables essentially require you to share a table. You can sit two seats down from the woman of your choice and easily strike up a conversation about where you're going.

Now that I think about it, my layover in Philadelphia yesterday would have been a great place to meet women as well. I was there around lunchtime when the food court in the US Airways terminal was jam-packed. Because all of the tables were small and couldn't accommodate more than one or two people, there wasn't an empty table to be found. After having to wake up so early, I wasn't in a particularly talkative mood, so I just took my food back to the gate. Now that I think about it, however, that would have been a great opportunity to approach a beautiful woman who was eating by herself and ask if I could pull up a chair. As crowded as the food court was, it would have been rude for a woman (or anyone for that matter) to decline a request to sit with her. And besides, who wouldn't want some company in a room – or entire airport – full of strangers when she or he has some down time?

2. Use the built-in opening line!

Steve and I, in *Make Every Girl Want You*™, discussed how to approach women and strike up a conversation. We discussed the importance of beginning with an open-ended question (preferably about her) and the importance of following up her response with a short remark of your own. We relayed the pattern of successful introductory conversation and emphasized the intangibles, including reticence, confidence, enthusiasm, eye contact, and the appropriate attitude to project. When meeting women in an airport, use the built-in introductory line: "So, where are you headed?" Asking this question serves three purposes:

1) It provides the initial icebreaker that you need. Given that you're in an airport, it's appropriate and natural to inquire about her travel plans. Even if she does pick up on the fact that you're hitting on her, she should be comfortable realizing that you're a Nice Guy, rather than a player who is going to ask her to join the Mile High Club.

2) It lends itself to a natural follow-up: "Oh, are you visiting there, or is that where you're from?"

3) The follow-up question will tell you where she lives so you know whether or not this is something worth pursuing.

For example, just now when I met Erica, she told me that she's going to Norfolk for Memorial Day weekend to visit her brother who's getting back into town after being stationed on the *U.S.S. Harry Truman.* She's going there for the ship's homecoming celebration. Discovering this information naturally led me to follow up by asking, "Oh, do you live in New York City?" It's unfortunate that she replied, "Yeah, I live in Brooklyn," because I live in a suburb of Norfolk. I wish she lived down there and was returning home, rather than up here.

3. Meeting women in an airport works better in your hometown

Here's an obvious point: You're likely to be more successful meeting dateable women in your home airport than when you're traveling somewhere else. If you're in a major airport or a hub, then I suppose that many of the women there merely have a layover and are neither from your city nor visiting your city. But I suspect that somewhere between 30-50% of the women you'd meet in your home airport actually live in or around your city. Regardless, using the opening question I suggested above will allow you to easily discover if this woman lives in your home city and if it's worth pursuing further contact with her.

Now that I've figured this out, I guess that chatting with women in LaGuardia today is pretty pointless, though I suppose that it's good practice for next time.

And let me tell you, there was a next time . . .

A few weeks after meeting Erica at LaGuardia, I met another woman at the airport – this time with more success! While sitting on the airplane, I wrote the following:

"I'm sitting on a plane to Charlotte right now, typing this about a woman who's sitting three rows behind me. I can't wait until we land in Charlotte so I can talk to her again!

I initially struck up a conversation with her in the ticket line at the US Airways ticket counter in the Newport News-Williamsburg Airport. Given that only two flights were scheduled to depart from this small airport within the next few hours, I knew there was a pretty high probability that she would be on my flight.

For some reason, the line at the airport was incredibly long, but I can't complain. We ended up getting to chat for about fifteen minutes while standing in line, and I found out that her name is Isabel. She's a beautiful woman from Venezuela. Following the advice from *Make Every Girl Want You*™, I was a perfect Nice Guy and showed a lot of interest in her. I didn't interrogate her, offered up some information about myself, and made great eye contact. Oh, yeah – and I told her how amazingly beautiful her smile is! Trust me, it is.

I made sure that I wasn't overly aggressive. I didn't ask for her contact info. Once I knew that she was on my flight and I'd have another opportunity to speak with her, I realized that I could turn this into a Moderately-Inviting Environment. She was ahead of me in line, and once she got past the ticket counter, she was off to the gate.

I went through security, proceeded straight to the gate, and grabbed a seat. I looked around for her. She wasn't there yet, so I took out a book and started reading. About twenty-five minutes later, I heard, 'Hey, John – you won't believe what just happened to me!'

I looked up and saw Isabel, who ran up and took the seat beside me. She then started telling me about how her bag had gotten searched because security mistook the bottle of Vodka in her luggage for explosives. They took the bottle out, opened the cap, and even started sniffing the Vodka.

Isabel was talking a mile a minute, laughing as she told the story. Her emotion (which wasn't all that different from my own) was a mixture of fear, shock, and exuberance. There was only one thought going through my mind the entire time: Thirty minutes ago, we didn't know each other from the other fifty people sitting in front of Gate 4. Yet, because I struck up a conversation with Isabel at the ticket counter, she ran up to me and couldn't wait to tell me her story! I think that officially makes us friends.

Now Isabel is sitting three rows behind me (we probably could have switched seats so we could sit next to each other, but I was so excited to write this chapter that I didn't want to sit next to her on the plane). Honestly, all I can think about is the fact that Isabel and I will get to chat again when we land at the Charlotte airport in about twenty minutes.

Isabel already asked me to wait for her when we land in Charlotte. Maybe we'll grab lunch if she has enough time before her next flight. Sure, things like this have happened to me dozens of times since I've been a Nice Guy, but I still can't get over it whenever it happens. It still amazes me how an hour ago I didn't know this woman, and now she wants me to wait for her in the Charlotte airport.

Sure, we're going in different directions from there, but as we're walking through the terminal, I plan to ask for her e-mail address. While we were standing in line together, I learned that she loves to salsa dance and told her that I'd love for her to give me some lessons. As per the instructions of *Make Every Girl Want You*™, I'll make sure that I ask for her e-mail address so she can teach me how to salsa dance sometime when we get back to Virginia Beach!

Let this be a testament to the power of striking up a conversation when you're in a place, such as an airport, where you find yourself surrounded by total strangers. A simple conversation can create a bond – maybe even a spark – between the two of you instantly."

Gyms

I just completed an interview for an article in *Men's Health* about meeting women at the gym, and I figured that this would make great material for my new book. As guys who want to make ourselves attractive to women – and stay healthy, of course – many of us go to the gym several times a week. Given the significant amount of time that we spend sweating on the treadmill and pumping a little iron, it makes sense to multi-task by meeting women while working out.

The first thing to keep in mind when meeting women at the gym is that you're in a Moderately-Inviting Environment (as introduced in the chapter "Getting Started: How to Meet Women" of *Make Every Girl Want You*™). What this means is that while women aren't at the gym specifically to meet guys, they're also not opposed to meeting guys there. As long as you approach the situation properly, you're not that big of a distraction to them.

As with any Moderately-Inviting Environment, the trick to meeting women at the gym is to avoid coming on too strong. Keep in mind that you will probably see this woman on multiple occasions. If you seem overly aggressive, you'll only end up scaring her away.

The easiest way to meet a particular woman at the gym is to work in with her on a machine. Simply wait until she has just begun using a machine, walk up, and ask, "Do you mind if I work in?" You can then use any of the standard questions from the Appendix to get the conversation rolling.

Often, I see women at the gym wearing clothes that make a great topic of conversation. For example, a woman might wear a shirt with a university name or sorority letters on it or gym shorts that are branded by a well-known ski apparel manufacturer. When you pick up on this sort of minutiae, it becomes easy to start a conversation by asking a question such as, "Oh, did you go to Ohio State?" Or you might say, "I noticed your shorts – are you a big skier?"

In the Ohio State example, if you learn that she attended Ohio State, you can follow up with these questions:

> "What did you major in?"
> "What brought you to <city you're presently in>?"
> "How did you like the school?"

And if she didn't go to Ohio State, you can follow up with these questions:

> "Are you from Ohio?"
> "Did you go to school around here?"
> "Oh, where'd you get the shirt from?"

In the ski-clothing example, you could follow up with questions such as:

> "How many times have you been skiing?"
> "Are you an expert?"
> "Where are some of your favorite places to ski?"
> "How old were you when you first learned how to ski?"

As this list of follow-up questions suggests, you should have no problem finding something to talk about as long as you make the effort to notice things about the woman's attire – or the machine she's using, the magazine she's reading, or any number of other context clues, as we call them in *Make Every Girl Want You*™. Remember, of course, to always offer up something about yourself in between asking questions so that you don't sound too nosy.

All of this being said, don't allow yourself to become overconfident (or what she'll construe as aggressive) and think that you should ask for her contact information the first time you're talking with her unless this is a woman you rarely see at the gym. If you're not overly aggressive the first time you chat with her, she's more likely to become comfortable around you. Plus, if she's someone you've seen there a few times, then you can probably assume that you'll see her around again, enabling you to establish a connection with her.

During the introductory conversation, make sure to get her name. That way you can make sure to always address her by name in the future since you're likely to run into each other there again. It is also essential that you remember any vital pieces of information that she relays to you. Go into the locker room and write them down if you have to.

When you follow all of these guidelines, you will be able to walk right up to her and strike up a conversation the next time you see her at the gym. If you think she may not remember you, perhaps because your first conversation was brief, try working in with her on a machine again. However, heed this word of caution: It's probably best not to work in with her on a machine more than once on any given day unless, of course, you want her to think that you have stalker tendencies. Obviously, if you have any interest in pursuing things with this woman, you don't want to give her that impression.

The second time I speak with someone, I like to initiate the conversation by saying, "Hey, <name>, right?" For example, "Hey, Veronica, right?" That way you can show her that you remember her name, which a woman will appreciate because it suggests that you're genuinely interested in her as a person. By phrasing your introduction as if you're uncertain whether you've gotten her name correct, you alleviate any awkwardness in the conversation if she has forgotten your name.

If that's the case, the woman will usually respond, "Yeah, it's Veronica. I'm sorry – what was your name again?" Don't be offended. If she's a beautiful woman, she probably gets approached by men all of the time.

During your second conversation, make sure you bring up some past piece of information that she mentioned. If, for example, a woman tells you that she's just taking a study break to come to the gym and mentions that she's studying for med school finals, then be sure to ask her how her exams went the next time you see her. And, of course, always remember to use the standard Nice Guy rules of conversation, such as making strong eye contact.

Once you've done all of this, follow the standard procedure that we presented in *Make Every Girl Want You*™ for getting a woman's contact info. As a refresher, we advise you to establish a couple of mutual interests through conversation. At the end of the conversation, ask for her contact info for the purpose of participating in an activity of mutual interest.

By watching Oscar at the gym, I've learned that waiting until you've spoken to the woman in question on a few different occasions at the gym tends to pay off. As you might expect, Oscar is very social at the gym. When Oscar strikes up a conversation with someone new, I've noticed that he never asks for her contact info during the introductory conversation. Oscar has the aptitude to realize that one brief chat isn't enough to warrant a woman giving out her contact info. Oscar knows that he'll inevitably run into her a couple more times in the next few weeks, so he patiently waits until they've had a couple more conversations before asking for her contact info. After she's had a few great conversations with Oscar, the woman is not only willing to give Oscar her contact info but is actually *eager* to do so when he requests it.

My friend Sheila's account of how she and her husband met confirms that patience pays off. As Sheila recalls:

> "Rick approached me one day in the gym. We had seen each other there a few times, and I guess we both kind of recognized each other. One day, he worked in with me on the leg curl machine.
>
> I was wearing some Burton pants, and he asked me if I like to ski. I am actually not much of a skier, but we ended up chatting about sports and outdoor activities in general. I mentioned that I love to run, and so did he.
>
> The conversation that day was short, but he kept working in with me on the leg curl every time we were at the gym. You'd think he could've at least chosen a different machine each time so that I couldn't tell that he was doing it intentionally!

During our fourth conversation, he finally asked for my e-mail address so we could go running together sometime. I was so glad that he *finally* asked; I was beginning to wonder if he would ever make the move! But I guess it's good that he was patient because I would've been a little sketched out if he asked for my e-mail address after our first short conversation. We hit it off from there, and I guess you could say that the rest is history now that we're happily married!"

As Sheila revealed, Rick used the standard no-pressure approach that we introduced in *Make Every Girl Want You*™. He discovered a mutual interest (running), told Sheila that he's always looking for someone to go running with, and eventually asked for her e-mail address.

If you're meeting someone at the gym, it's quite possible that the two of you share some other common athletic interest, such as running, skiing, tennis, racquetball, or hiking. If this is the case, you've got a great excuse to ask for her contact info! I remember that the gym I used to belong to had racquetball courts. If I had ever met a girl there who loved to play racquetball, I would've definitely asked for her contact info so we could meet at the gym sometime to play racquetball. A great way to follow up our game would have been to grab lunch together.

Cruises

I'm on a cruise in the Caribbean right now and, oh man, is this the place to meet women! There was an abundance of gorgeous women lounging by the pool this afternoon. I talked to a few of them, which inspired me to come back to my cabin and write a chapter about meeting women on cruise ships.

I suppose much of this advice would work in basically any vacation hotspot. However, because the cruise ship itself is self-contained, I think a cruise provides an added advantage over other vacation spots. Right now, I'm onboard with two thousand other people. I know that the women I was chatting with out by the pool earlier are somewhere on this ship right now. Sure, one may be in the casino right now, one may be eating dinner, one may be getting dressed, and one may be grabbing a drink. But they're all somewhere on this ship. Odds are, I'll run into at least one of them later this evening while carousing around this city on water.

I've actually been on a few cruises, and here's what I've learned about women on cruise ships: About half of the women on this ship are probably here with a guy. But most of the other women on this ship are probably here with a female friend, or better yet, a group of female friends. Those are the women you want to start chatting with. It is important to keep in mind that a cruise ship is a Moderately-Inviting Environment. Because most people there don't really know anyone on the ship, passengers tend to be very open to meeting people, particularly during the first couple of days.

Recognizing that they're in an anonymous environment hundreds or thousands of miles from their daily lives, women on cruises often leave many of their inhibitions back on land. These women are often just looking to have a good time and enjoy their vacation. One of my friends Alyssa had this to say about her mindset while on vacation with her girlfriends:

> "When I'm on vacation, all the rules change! I mean, when I'm at home, anything you do gets talked about by all of your friends, much less the entire community. But when you're on vacation, with only your good friends, whatever

happens stays there! Now, I'm not saying we're bad girls or anything, but yeah – we do like to have our fun! And the best part about a vacation is meeting guys who live on the other side of the country – or globe – and not having to worry about any stories surfacing once I return home. It's like taking a week out of life, with no repercussions! That's why vacations are so great!!"

With this in mind, let's now discuss the best spots to meet women on a cruise ship so that you can maximize your ship's love boat potential. The best place to meet women has to be out on deck. Typically, most single women on the ship wake up fairly early in the morning and head out on deck to lay by the pool and tan. Working to perfect their tans, the most beautiful women are often the first ones out there.

I got up at 8 AM this morning despite being hung-over and exhausted. Getting a prime seat right next to one of the most beautiful women on this ship definitely made it worth it, though. I brought a book to read – and my patience – with me. After about fifteen minutes of reading, I struck up a conversation with her and learned that her name is Amy and that she's currently working on her Master's degree in biology at the University of California.

I chatted with Amy for a while until she left the deck to take a yoga class. Afterwards, I discovered how easy it is to network with women around the pool area. For example, you can hop in the pool to cool off and grab a seat somewhere else when you get out. Or you can stay in the pool and meet women as they get in the water to cool off. Doing this, I met quite a few women by the pool in the span of a few short hours.

The many buffets on a cruise ship are another great place to meet women. Although the dining rooms typically have assigned seating for dinner, the breakfast, lunch, and midnight buffets usually have open seating, which allows passengers to sit wherever they choose. This afternoon, I went to the lunch buffet right at 12:30 since I knew that all of the tables would be packed at that time. After getting a tray full of food, I conveniently found myself with no choice but to walk up to a table where two attractive women were seated and ask if I could sit with them. These two seniors at the University of Alabama gladly accepted, though they really didn't have much of a choice. There were no tables available, so it would have been impolite for them to deny me the seat.

The casino is also a great place to meet women on board a cruise ship. You can easily walk up to a woman, sit down next to her, and strike up a conversation, as long as she isn't too involved in whatever game she's playing. Try this by the slot machines; that way, the two of you can take your time and chat without holding up anyone else at the table.

Another great time to meet women on a cruise ship is just after dinner, around eight or nine o'clock. At this time, everyone is usually pretty full from dinner and isn't ready to start drinking and enjoying the nightlife yet. Women are often strolling around the ship as they walk off dinner and search for something to do. During this time, I often run into women out on deck and strike up a conversation.

And, of course, don't forget the obvious: Cruise ships have a number of bars and clubs in which you can easily approach women at night. I prefer, however, to meet women during the day when I can have a great, casual introductory conversation out by the pool. That way, they already know me and are happy to see me when I run into them later that night in a bar.

Another tip for those of you who will be cruising in the future: It's really important to meet women on the first day or two that you're on the ship. During the first day or two, you're typically at sea and spend all day on the ship, making it very easy to meet women. On subsequent days, however, your ship is often at port. If you haven't yet met women on the ship by that point, then you're on your own when you go ashore. On the other hand, if you spent the first day meeting women, as I did today, then you can make plans to go out on land with them during the next few days. For example, I have plans to head out to the beaches of Grand Cayman tomorrow with two sisters from Florida whom I met earlier today.

For those of you who have never been on a cruise before and are thinking of taking one, let me offer a bit of advice about choosing a cruise ship. It is important to choose your cruise line and ship appropriately. Each cruise line attracts a specific demographic. For example, some cruises are designated as "singles' cruises," which you might want to consider. I've never actually taken one of those and don't think it's necessary because I've always found plenty of single women on the cruises that I've taken. Disney cruises, meanwhile, are geared toward families with young children while Holland America seems to attract an older crowd. If you're a single man in your fifties or sixties, you may want to consider a cruise on a Holland America ship. If, however, you're in your twenties or thirties, you probably want to opt for a cruise line such as Carnival.

There are plenty of websites available that can point you in the right direction, or you can ask your travel agent for a recommendation on what cruise lines would be best suited for you. Once you do that, you'll be well on your way to discovering the wonders of the love boat firsthand.

Although you now know how to meet women in a variety of places, from bars to airports to the gym, we at The Nice Guys' Institute™ are constantly working on tips for meeting women in other environments. Please visit www.TheNiceGuysGuide.com to learn about our latest findings.

Visit the site often as we are constantly updating it with new content, including downloadable e-books and e-reports, audio tapes and CDs, and video cassettes and DVDs packed with our latest discoveries.

We also maintain information on our web site about upcoming coaching sessions, course offerings, and speaking engagements. Additionally, we encourage readers to e-mail us, either through our web site, or at TheNiceGuys@TheNiceGuysGuide.com. Finally, please also come by and sign up for our free newsletter to receive the hottest tips to help nice guys like you make themselves more attractive to women WITHOUT turning into jerks!

Chapter 4 – The Nice Guys' Guide™ to Online Dating

Without fail, at least one guy asks me for advice about online dating each time I teach a class. I have also received literally hundreds of e-mails asking me for advice on this subject. When we wrote *Make Every Girl Want You™*, the online dating phenomenon was just taking hold, so Steve and I didn't have much experience with it. Consequently, we didn't devote much attention to this important topic in our first book. Since then, however, online dating has become commonplace, and we at The Nice Guys' Institute™ have done a lot of research and testing on it, and continue to research the subject. You've waited long enough for guidance on this matter. So without further ado, I offer you the first official guide to meeting women online (with more advice to follow in the future!).

Currently, I am in the midst of a little online dating experiment of my own. Pretending to be an incredibly beautiful woman, I created a fake profile on Match.com in order to see what kind of responses I'd get from men. The responses have been incredible! It will take a while for me to sort through these responses, analyze them, and ask the opinions of my female friends, so there will be more information available even after this book goes to press. In order to ensure that you can stay abreast of the latest advice and news about online dating, I intend to post my findings in an online report on www.TheNiceGuysGuide.com as soon as they are available. If you're interested in getting the latest information on this rapidly evolving craze, please take a moment right now to visit www.TheNiceGuysGuide.com.

The rest of this chapter is dedicated to what I've learned so far from talking to my female friends and from the test profiles that I've created on sites such as Match.com. Much like in the world of offline dating, the male typically plays the role of pursuer in the world of online dating, while the woman waits to be pursued. For this reason, it would be ill-advised for you to simply create a profile and hope that some beautiful woman will e-mail you. The world of online dating just doesn't work that way. As a male, I have found that you have to take the initiative. In fact, it is nearly impossible to get a woman to respond to your profile on Match.com. It appears that women merely create their own profile and wait for guys to e-mail them, which apparently happens in droves. They then select a few e-mails, respond to them, and things evolve from there.

With this in mind, the first obvious step in your pursuit of online dating should be to pick an online dating website, set up an account, and create your profile. Honestly, you shouldn't spend too much time worrying about what you say in your profile because, as I said, women don't really browse Match.com and then e-mail the guys with the best profiles. I actually had the most success online when I kept my profile succinct. Because the first thing a woman will most likely see is your e-mail to her, you should focus most of your energy there rather than on your profile. Women have told me that you give yourself a rather sexy aura of mystery when you don't reveal much in the profile; they think that guys who write their entire life stories in their online profiles appear desperate.

When I asked my friend Sarah about online profiles, she offered me the following insight:

> "My biggest pet peeve about meeting guys online is that everyone feels the need to reveal so much about himself up front. Actually, some guys write their entire life stories in their profiles, and I have to be honest, my girlfriends and I have discussed this. When a guy does that, it makes him look really desperate.
>
> All of my girlfriends and I agree that there's something alluring about the mystery of getting to know someone in person. The best part about meeting a new guy is those first few dates when you find out so much about each other.
>
> A word of advice for guys: Keep your online profiles short, and don't reveal too much to us in your first few e-mails. Keep us wondering and give us something to look forward to when we meet you in person."

Don't think that this means that you shouldn't bother filling out the profile at all. When women receive an intriguing e-mail from you, they will go straight to your profile to check you out. So definitely make sure that you take a few minutes to fill out your profile; just don't waste too much time here.

Here's another thing to keep in mind when writing your profile: Most guys go on and on about their hobbies in their online profiles. While it's important to mention some of your hobbies, it's even more important to mention some of your character traits. Take the time to relay to women, for instance, that you're very honest, or tell them what you're passionate about. If this is the case, you might say that you're really close to your family or that you've often been told you're really sensitive. Conveying emotional character traits such as these can score you a lot of points with a woman.

Additionally, you *must* post a picture if you want women to grace you with a response. Thinking that any woman who truly wants to get to know me won't care what I look like, I tried omitting a picture. Bad idea. Let's be honest: you're only going to e-mail women who have their photo posted online, which means that you should only expect a response back if you have posted your picture as well. Women who have taken the time – and the risk – to post their photo online will view you as cowardly or lazy if you don't take the same time and risk to post your own photo.

Once you've posted your profile and picture, the real fun begins. Start browsing the website, do some searches, and find some women who interest you. Just don't get hung up on any one woman. You have to accept that the odds of any one woman responding to you aren't that great. Remember, depending on which online dating site you're using and which city you live in, each woman may get dozens of e-mails a day. Getting hung up on a particular woman just isn't a wise move if you want to ensure that you experience the dating aspect of online dating.

When browsing the profiles at online dating sites, you'll probably notice that about two or three of the women are just strikingly gorgeous. These women are typically hot enough that they could be models, even though in almost all cases, they're not. If you've always wanted to date a model, don't get your hopes up that online dating is the way to go. In the offline world, I see women who are this beautiful on occasion – in bookstores, coffee shops, bars, or just out around town. Most of the time when I see them, they're not with guys. If I approach one of these women in a coffee shop, for example, there's usually not some other guy vying for her attention. Even though I am bothering her in this situation as Steve and I discussed in *Make Every Girl Want You*™, the fact that there's no immediate competition means that I'll get a fair shot with her.

In the online world, however, the exact opposite is true. When a girl is this hot (or her picture makes her look this hot), then every guy with an online subscription will be e-mailing her. I've tried numerous different e-mails and a variety of approaches, and I still have yet to be graced with a response from one of these model-hot women. Even when I used a fake picture of a male model in my profile, not one of these women responded.

Having flashbacks to my college days when I couldn't get women to give me the time of day, I decided to conduct a little experiment. I wanted to see what it would be like to be a hot girl, so I created a fake profile, using a picture of a model from a clothing catalog. I posted the ad at night and then went to bed. By noon the following morning, I had already received fifty responses from guys. During the first week after I posted that picture, I received an average of forty to fifty e-mails a day from guys.

I wanted to see if all women receive this many responses or if I received that many because I had made my "female self" so hot. So, I repeated the experiment, but I used a picture of a girl who's pretty but not model-hot instead. Over that next week, I only received about twenty responses per day to that profile. The conclusion? In the online world, every guy goes after the drop-dead gorgeous women. The odds of your e-mail even being read are close to non-existent. Now, I'm not telling you to chase after ugly or below-average women here. I'm just saying that if you want to have any luck in the online dating world, it's more fruitful to focus on pretty women than on model-hot women.

Once you've chosen a few pretty women to send e-mails to, the next step is to actually e-mail them. Don't forget to include something in the subject line. Remember, the subject is the first thing that the woman will see, so the words you choose for your subject heading may determine the recipient's first impression of you. Let's be honest, you need to make yourself stand out among a couple dozen guys. The more creative the subject that you come up with, the better. It's even OK to put something a little outrageous in the subject just as long as it's not offensive.

The body of the e-mail, though, is what ultimately counts. Here are some guidelines for the body of the e-mail: First of all, make it a point to say that you're a little nervous or hesitant about meeting women online. Most women tell me that they are very apprehensive about meeting guys online after some of the crazy stories they've heard, and my female friends have told me that it's very reassuring to hear that a guy is trying this for the first time as well.

Since a woman's biggest fear is meeting a stalker, crazed lunatic, or rapist on the internet, I've often found it helpful to say in the initial e-mail that I'm new to this online dating thing and am just trying it out. By illuminating your shared apprehension, you can (subtly) convey to her that you're just as normal as she is. When I asked my friend Natalie her thoughts about meeting guys online, she revealed:

> "I'm definitely weirded-out about meeting guys on the internet. My biggest fear is that the guy on the other end of my computer is some stalker or a guy who surfs online dating sites to find his next rape victim. I just feel a lot better when I know that the guy I'm e-mailing is new to this online dating thing.
>
> I've met some guys who openly admit that they've been on Match.com for a year and a half and still haven't met anyone. Knowing that just gives me a bad vibe about the guy. It just makes me really, really uncomfortable to know that I'm e-

mailing some guy who's sitting there all day long – and all year long – stalking women online."

Additionally, if you're new to the area, indicate that in your e-mail. I asked my friend Paige why women feel better when a guy indicates that he's just moved to the area. She thought about it for a few seconds before replying:

> "I don't really know. But I know when a guy e-mails me on Match.com and says that he just recently moved to Chicago, I feel less intimidated by the whole thing. I feel like he's saying, 'Hey, I'm new to the city, and I don't really know many people here. You look like a friendly face, so I just wanted to shoot you an e-mail.'
>
> I'm sure that 99% of the time, the guy has actually lived in Chicago his entire life and is saying that he's new to town just so he doesn't sound like a loser, but I don't know, it's still kind of reassuring."

The next thing to remember when writing that introductory e-mail is to compliment the woman. I prefer to compliment her twice actually, once on her physical beauty and once on a non-physical attribute. Sure, the physical compliment can be a little tricky since you've typically only seen one tiny photo of her online. However, I've found that you can usually find some feature, such as a woman's beautiful eyes or her pretty smile, to compliment her on. In some cases, I've simply told a woman that I thought she was beautiful.

I'm sure that a lot of women receive physical compliments online, so I always make sure to convey a non-physical compliment as well. I usually find something in her profile and compliment her on that. For example, I might tell her how impressed I am that she's so dedicated to horseback riding or that I think it's really cool that she went hiking in the Alps last summer. I've found that just by picking out a character trait from a profile and telling the woman how impressed you are by it, you can really set yourself apart from other men.

The next step is to offer up some information about yourself. You typically don't need to include a physical description of yourself because when the woman visits your profile online, she'll see the physical description that you've already filled out. Speaking of which, make sure that you are honest and that everything you say in both your profile and your initial e-mail is true and accurate. There's nothing more disappointing to a woman than meeting someone in person and realizing that he lied about himself. Let's be honest. You would not be pleased if a woman told you that she was tall, blond, 29, and in med school, and then you met her and found out that she wasn't even out of middle school and wasn't blond or tall. So don't think that you can lie to a woman just to get a date with her and then expect that she'll realize what a great personality you have despite the fact that you blatantly lied to her. Basing your entire relationship (what little of it there is initially) on a lie is doomed to backfire. As my friend Emily relates:

> "I met this guy Jim online. He was very sweet in his e-mails, and he looked so hot in his picture . . . But when I met him, I realized that that wasn't even his picture. He looked nothing like the guy in the picture, and he was two inches shorter than the height he had listed in the profile!
>
> Needless to say, as soon as I saw him, I realized that he had tricked me, which put me in a really sour mood. So twenty minutes into the date, I went into the

bathroom and called one of my friends, told her what had happened, and asked her to call and fake an emergency in five minutes so I could get out of the date. Five minutes later, my phone rang, and that's the last I ever saw of Jim.

The thing is, he wasn't a bad-looking guy; I just wish he hadn't lied to me about his physical description. The fact that he did just showed me how insecure he was. It's a shame, too, because he wasn't bad looking, and his e-mails were really sweet."

While it's important to be honest about your identity, there are some things that are better left unsaid in the world of online dating. Inevitably, you will go out with a woman whom you met online, and she will ask how many other women you e-mailed. If you want to see her again, you do *not* want her to think that you e-mailed a few dozen women (although, as I've stated, the only way you'll get a response from a woman or two is if you take the time to fire off e-mails to a few dozen women!). When the woman inevitably asks how many women you e-mailed, you don't need to lie and tell her she was the only one. However, you should probably refrain from telling her if you had to e-mail dozens of women before one responded. You can usually answer this touchy question by tying your response into a compliment. You could say something along the lines of, "Well, I e-mailed a few women, but you had by far the prettiest smile, so I was really excited when you e-mailed me back."

I've given you lots of do's and don'ts for writing that first e-mail, but you may still be wondering exactly what a well-composed introductory e-mail might look like. Here's a sample e-mail that my friend Jorge sent to a woman on Match.com that elicited an almost-immediate response:

"Hey! I'm a little nervous about meeting people online, but I recently moved to the D.C. area & don't know many people here so I figured I'd give it a try. Anyway, your profile caught my eye. You are astonishingly beautiful & I'm guessing you get dozens of responses a day, so I'll keep mine short! What caught my eye - more than just your beauty - is your ambition & dedication. I'm very impressed that you knew what you wanted to do at such a young age and went after it!

Alright, a little about me. I really like the outdoors, and I am always going hiking, playing tennis, or going out on a friend's boat. I'm a laid-back guy who gets along with pretty much everybody. I've always had a lot of friends, both guys & girls, and consider honesty the most important trait in a good friend. That's enough for now. I hope to hear from you soon. Have a good afternoon!"

Here's the response he received a few minutes later:

"Jorge, hey, your e-mail was such a great way to end my day! I wouldn't say I get *dozens* of responses from Match.com, but yours was among several this afternoon – and the only one I felt compelled to reply to. You're the most sincere guy to e-mail me so far!

So, more about me: I also just moved to the area and want to meet new people. My co-workers are great, but I also need to have a life outside of work, right? I'm also a little sketched-out about this whole meeting people online thing, so much so that I usually hide my profile. It's only on days when I'm feeling especially risqué that I un-hide it for people to see :) I've been on Match.com for about a month now, though, and nothing terrible has come of it. Keep your fingers crossed . . .

Let's see . . . I LOVE the beach, ice cream, sunrise, running (I'm running my first marathon in 20 days!!!), and pretty much anything associated with summer. I'm looking forward to lots of sunshine and snow-free forecasts! I love my job, my family, and my car. I don't want to give away all of my secrets now, but I hope these were enough to convince you that I might be a 'quality' girl that you'd like to get to know better. When you have a chance, tell me more about you: your job, your musical tastes, anything! Oh yeah, when I checked out your profile, I saw that you're a Taurus, so happy birthday!

Looking forward to hearing from you . . . Jackie :)"

So, what happens when you master the skill of writing the introductory e-mail, and after sending a few e-mails out to some women, one actually e-mails you back? What next? Now it's time to exchange some more e-mails with her, learn a little about each other, and really get a dialogue going between the two of you. Whatever you do, don't jump the gun. Don't invite her to meet you somewhere yet. Approach the e-mails much the same you would with a woman you met in person, as outlined in the "Getting Contact Info and Making Future Contact" chapter of *Make Every Girl Want You™*. Ask her some questions from the Appendix, and for every question you ask her, offer up some information about yourself (such as your answer to the question you're asking).

Exchanging a few e-mails back and forth in this manner will accomplish a couple of things. First of all, you'll learn a lot about each other, which will enable you to get to know her better and help in planning future dates. Second, you'll build rapport and make her feel more comfortable around you. Here's a sample second e-mail that Jorge sent to Jackie after she responded to his initial e-mail:

> "Hey, Jackie! I finally got a free minute to write back during lunch. First off, thanks for the b-day wishes! You actually nailed the day – my b-day was yesterday! So thank you very much!
>
> I'm glad to hear that family is important to you – it's very important to me as well. My parents & brother both live down in Florida, which means I can go down & visit occasionally (or make them come up here!). My parents are celebrating their 37th anniversary this winter (can you believe it?!). Do you have any siblings? Where does your family live?
>
> As for me, I really like my job. I work for CIO (yes, those wonderful commercials) in the IT department. It's challenging, and I struggled a bit when I joined, but since then, I've really started to enjoy it. So, where do you work ? That's great that you get along well with your co-workers – mine are pretty cool, too.
>
> Glad to see you are also a big fan of the beach. I actually grew up on the Jersey shore and LOVE the beach! Ah, I miss

those days at the Jersey shore. Where are
you from originally?

Alright, I'm gonna go grab some lunch.
Have a good afternoon, Jackie!"

Now the real fun begins. After you've exchanged
a few e-mails back and forth like Jorge and Jackie,
invite the woman in question to meet you for a drink or
coffee. When I asked my female friends, they
overwhelmingly preferred to meet a guy whom they've
met online either in a coffee shop or at a bar since there
would be plenty of other people around in case the guy
turned out to be a little shady. So, whatever you decide
to do, make sure to meet her in a public place.
Remember, she isn't yet certain that you're not a
stalker, lunatic, or rapist, so she will probably be very
hesitant to meet up with you anyplace where there
aren't a lot of other people around.

On the same note, you shouldn't treat the initial
meeting as a first date. Think of it as more of an
introductory date. You're just two people getting to
know each other a little better at a bar or coffee shop.
Keep in mind that she will probably be extremely
nervous, and you might be as well. After you've chatted
for a while, simply tell her that you enjoyed meeting
her, that you've had a great time, and say good night.
Do not invite her to go anywhere else that evening.
Likewise, do not try to make physical contact with her,
and definitely don't try to kiss her goodnight. Save that
for the first real date. Remember, the point of this initial
meeting is just to get to know each other a little better
in a relaxed environment.

So now the two of you have met on this
introductory date, and she realizes that you are a
normal, nice guy and someone whom she enjoys being
around. Where do you go from here? I've found that it is
a good idea to shoot her an e-mail the following day,
reiterating how much you enjoyed meeting her. I'll
usually bring up something from the conversation,

such as wishing her good luck with her presentation that afternoon. Then I'll wait for her to e-mail me back.

After she's written me back, I'll usually reply and propose that we go out on a date. Keep in mind that this will now be your actual first date; be mindful of the advice that Steve and I offer on everything from planning the date to how to behave on the date in the "Getting Contact Info and Making Future Contact" chapter of *Make Every Girl Want You*™. At this point, it's just like any other date, so follow the instructions in *Make Every Girl Want You*™ and have fun!

Out-of-Town Online Dating

One of the hottest new crazes that I've been hearing about is Out-of-Town Online Dating. This is for people, such as consultants, who travel for their job and return back to that same city all week long, week after week. Quite frequently, a guy tells me something like:

> "Hey, John. I'm a consultant, and I work really long hours. I live in New York City, but my project is in Atlanta right now. I'll be there for the next year. Since I work really long hours, I don't have much time to go out and try to meet women. But I would really love to meet someone down in Atlanta, someone I can take out to dinner after a long day of work (at the company's expense!), someone who will make me look forward to being out-of-town all week.
>
> Is there any easy way to do this? I mean – I've thought about using online dating sites, but I'm not sure how that works. Do I lie in my profile and say that I live in Atlanta? Otherwise it only searches for

women in New York City. Have you heard
of guys having success with this before?"

Taken together, the combination of a growing
online dating trend and an increasing number of people
whose jobs require frequent travel produced a new
mode of dating – out-of-town online dating. Don't get
the wrong idea. Out-of-town online dating is not at all
about one night stands. It's not intended for guys who
spend every night in a different city and are just looking
for a quick fling in each town. Rather, out-of-town
online dating was designed to enable guys (and women)
whose jobs take them out-of-town to the same city each
week to build a relationship with someone in that city.

Now that you know what out-of-town online
dating is, here are some rules of thumb to keep in
mind: First, because you have limited free time in that
city with which to meet new women, the best means to
starting an out-of-town relationship is to use an online
dating site, such as Match.com. Follow the standard
online dating rules that I presented earlier in this
chapter in order to meet a few women and initiate a
casual e-mail dialogue. As with using an online dating
site to meet a woman in your hometown, keep in mind
that it is very important to be patient and take the time
to build rapport by exchanging a few e-mails before you
actually meet. Thus, if you're going to be in Dallas next
week for only a couple of weeks, it's probably too late to
meet someone using this method. However, if you're in
the first month of a three-month project, then you can
begin this process now. In about two to three weeks,
you will probably get to meet a woman or two in person
for the first time! Don't forget, though, that women are
very skeptical of these online dating sites and tend to
be overly cautious. As with any other online dating
scenario, you should meet and stay in public places the
first few times the two of you get together in order for
her to become more comfortable around you.

Here's another important rule to follow: Be
completely honest about your situation. Just as you

shouldn't pretend that you're tall, dark, and rich if you're not, you should *not* pretend that you live in that city. Explain to the woman that you live in another city but that you're in her city every week for business and are interested in meeting someone. Tell her, for instance, that you spend more time in Atlanta during the week than you do in New York, and so you've realized that it makes more sense to meet someone in Atlanta.

Likewise, you need to be honest about your intentions. If your project is coming to an end in three months, and you're really just looking for a three-month fling, say that! As I peruse women's profiles on Match.com, I notice that there are quite a few women on there who say that they're not looking for anything serious themselves, so don't fool yourself into thinking that it's necessary to lie about your intentions to get a woman to go out with you. Whatever the situation is, you're both more likely to enjoy each other's company and have a little fun when honesty provides the foundation for your relationship.

Also, remember to pace yourself in your out-of-town online dating relationship. At some point, you're likely to decide that you want her to visit your home city, probably over a weekend. This is a great thing to do . . . eventually. A word of advice though: Don't make the offer too prematurely. I've seen quite a few guys meet a woman, go out with her two or three times, and then invite her to come visit for the weekend. While this is a nice gesture, remember that there's a big difference between merely getting along with someone for a few hours at a time on a weeknight, and having her come stay for an entire weekend. I've seen many budding relationships fail because the couple prematurely tried to spend a weekend together before they were ready. With that in mind, make sure that the two of you are ready to spend the weekend together before you invite her to visit you on your turf. But, most importantly, have fun! I've heard many success stories from guys who have met great women through Out-of-Town

Online Dating. If you invest a little time and effort into e-mailing women, you could be next!

Part II The Nice Guys' Guide™ to Approaching Women

In the "Approaching Women" chapter of Make Every Girl Want You™, Steve and I introduced the distinct pattern to successful introductory conversation between a male and a female and provided a sample introductory conversation with analysis. In Part II of The Nice Guys' Guide™, I will offer further advice on approaching women, engaging a woman in conversation, and maintaining that conversation long enough to get her contact info that we at The Nice Guys' Institute™ have recently discovered.

Chapter 5 – The Nice Guys' Guide™ to Conveying Interest in a Conversation

Experts often say that the majority of communication is non-verbal and that it's not so much what you say but how you say it. We're told that everything from your tone to your body language to your expression sends a message to the other person, much more so than your words do.

In *Make Every Girl Want You*™, Steve and I discussed how to approach women and start a conversation. We discussed the importance of beginning with an open-ended question and following up her response with a short remark of your own. We described the pattern of successful introductory conversation and emphasized the intangibles, including reticence, confidence, enthusiasm, eye contact, and the appropriate attitude to project.

Yet, I've noticed that many guys still don't properly communicate with women even after I teach them how to converse with the opposite sex. These guys tell me that they do everything that Steve and I suggested in *Make Every Girl Want You*™. They ask questions, they listen to the woman's answer, they offer up a short response about themselves, and they ask further questions of the woman. But when I observe these guys in action, they're sending non-verbal signals to the woman that convey that they really don't care about what she has to say. To help these guys out in their quest for success with women, I've decided to dedicate a chapter in this book to conveying interest in a conversation. The conversational rules that I outline in this chapter serve to enhance your skills at conveying interest in what another person is saying, be it a woman whom you're interested in, your girlfriend's mother, a male co-worker, or anyone else whom you might find yourself having a conversation with on any given day.

1. Face the Woman

I've observed a lot of guys who will turn and talk to a woman with their face, but their bodies face a different direction. Unfortunately, this isn't going to cut it. Just as your TV would think that you didn't care about the football game on the screen if you kept looking out the window and up at the ceiling (like that would ever happen!), a woman is going to assume that you're not interested in what she has to say if you're not facing her. In order to convey interest in a conversation, then, it's important to face the woman. When you turn and face someone with your body, it sends the signal, "Hey, I'm interested in talking to you."

Likewise, if you're seated, lean forward while you're talking to the person. When most people are seated, they tend to lean back, probably because reclining is more comfortable. However, this sends the wrong signal to your conversational partner by suggesting that you're withdrawn from the conversation.

I've learned from watching Oscar that leaning forward is essential to convey interest in the conversation – and person – at hand. When he is seated, Oscar usually starts the conversation by sitting upright. During the conversation, he slowly leans in toward the person. I've noticed that by the end of the conversation, whomever Oscar is chatting with is usually leaning in toward him as well! The way that Oscar draws people into the conversation by leaning in toward them while speaking seems almost hypnotic at times. I used to think this was just part of Oscar's mystique, but Oscar is simply leaning in little by little to express deeper interest in the conversation. Truth be told, practically every other guy I've observed tends to lean back and slouch when he's having a conversation while seated.

2. Make Eye Contact

I'm always amazed – and disappointed – when I go out at night and observe other guys trying to pick up women. Most guys look at anything but the woman's eyes. They'll check out other women walking by, or they'll look at a woman's breasts. Sometimes they'll look at the bridge of her nose, her mouth, or her smile. I'll often catch guys watching the game on the TV above. On occasion, they might glance into the woman's eyes, but this is usually a fleeting glance. This, my friends, is a bad move on your part. You might as well tell the woman, "I really don't care what you have to say," because that's definitely the signal you're sending her with your body language. Part of the problem, I suspect, stems from the unfortunate fact that we as guys are never taught how to convey interest in a conversation. The vast majority of men that I come across – even men in their forties, fifties and sixties – don't yet know how to convey interest in a conversation. One of my friends Grace talks about her disgust with guys staring at her breasts:

> "Why do guys always stare at women's breasts? Do they think we can't tell?? Seriously! When you look right at a woman's breasts, we can tell! Look in our eyes – my eyes are up here. Please don't look down there, it's such a turn-off!"

Most women, on the other hand, seem to be cognizant of all of the important facets of relaying non-verbal interest in a conversation by the time they're teenagers. For instance, women recognize the importance of eye contact. In fact, most women consider the eyes to be the most communicative part of the body. One thing that's amazed me since I've become friends with a multitude of women is how women know the eye color of every guy they've ever met. Women will make comments, such as:

> "Oh, he has the most beautiful brown eyes."
> "The second I saw his bright blue eyes, he had me."
> "I've never seen hazel eyes more gorgeous than his."

Do you honestly think that eyes vary that drastically from person to person? Or that some guys have eyes that you'd describe as 'beautiful' or 'gorgeous'? Personally, I don't really think so. Sure, occasionally, I'll meet a guy whose eyes are extremely bright. For example, I have a male friend who has the brightest blue eyes. Because they really are a brighter shade of blue than any I've ever seen before, I can understand why women go crazy over his eyes.

But I've also observed other guys who my female friends think have gorgeous eyes, and in over 90% of these cases, I can't find anything distinctive about the guy's eyes. However, I have noticed something about these guys that distinguishes them from the rest of our gender. As far as I can tell, these guys have two things in common: they make intense eye contact when they talk, and they smile a lot. From this, I started to pick up on the importance of making strong eye contact and smiling.

I became convinced of the importance of these two non-verbal communication practices, however, through my own little experiment of sorts. For years, women have been telling me that Oscar has gorgeous eyes, and I can tell you first-hand: He doesn't. When I first started observing Oscar, I checked, and there was nothing special about Oscar's eyes! They looked exactly like mine. In fact, the only difference between my eyes and Oscar's was that Oscar made intense eye contact and smiled a lot. I had always wondered why women never said that I had beautiful eyes, so after noticing this difference between my eyes and Oscar's, I decided to make it a point to smile a lot and make intense eye contact. Almost immediately, I noticed that the more eye contact I made and the more that I smiled, the more women complimented me on my eyes! In fact, I now know when I haven't been making enough eye contact or smiling enough because I notice that it's been a while since I received my last compliment. If you make the effort to do these two things, women just might start telling their friends what beautiful eyes you have as well!

Simply making eye contact isn't enough, though. Make sure that you don't have shifty eyes like an acquaintance of mine, Jordan, who has a real problem with eye contact. Because Jordan can't focus his eyes in one position for more than a second, it's very unnerving to have a conversation with him. I'll look at Jordan's eyes and notice his eyes looking back at me. For a second, they'll glance at my left eye, then my right eye, then my nose, then my mouth, then my ear, then my chest, then my arm, then back to my left eye, then my cheek, and then back to my right eye. I'm sure he doesn't realize the negative message that he sends by doing this, and if I knew him better, I would talk to him about it.

The reason that Jordan's shifty eyes unnerve me is that this body language signals dishonesty and anxiety. In fact, notice how women have described Jordan, whom I find completely normal except for the eye issue:

> Amber: "Yeah, Jordan's a pretty shady guy."

> Julia: "The last time I was talking to him, I felt really nervous the whole time. I had nothing to be apprehensive about, but he just made me very nervous."

> Alissa: "Personally, I feel uncomfortable when I'm having a conversation with Jordan, so I always try to avoid talking to him alone."

> Amanda: "Oh, Jordan? He's very insecure from what I can tell."

> Mia: "You know, he's a nice guy. He just doesn't seem to have much confidence."

Again, there's nothing abnormal or bad about this guy, except for his eye issue, but his nervous eyes scare women away. He'd probably be quite popular with women if he could get over the eye problem. He's a bodybuilder, and I think any other guy with his body would be attracting more women than he would know what to do with.

While nervous eyes can be annoying, it is important to remember to break eye contact occasionally. As unnerving as it is for someone to avoid eye contact, it is equally unsettling when someone constantly stares at you without blinking or breaking eye contact. To ensure that you make eye contact at a frequency that doesn't freak out the person you're speaking to, it's a good idea to look into that person's eyes for about five to ten seconds while he or she is speaking and then look away for a second or two when there's a natural pause in the conversation. Then look back for another five or ten seconds while you're responding.

I've given you quite a bit of advice about what to do with your eyes to reassure a woman that you're interested in what she has to say, but occasionally, a guy will also ask me whether a woman is attracted to him if her eyes dilate while he's speaking to her. Personally, I don't have any proof of whether or not this is the case, but I did come across some information on the internet about this. Apparently, a person's pupils dilate (expand) when she sees something or someone that she is attracted to or likes. This is true both of a person they're attracted to and an object that they want. Apparently, for example, when a woman goes shopping and sees a dress that she really wants, her pupils expand. The same is probably true of guys when we see a car that we really like.

Yes, you probably can pay attention to a person's pupil size. If the pupils are dilated, then the person is possibly interested in you. I wouldn't rely too heavily on this, however, because there are other reasons why people's pupils dilate. For instance, drug use often causes your pupils to dilate. I would certainly hate to think that a girl was enjoying my company, when in actuality she's just high on crack. Another more common factor is the brightness of a room. In a very dark room, your pupils dilate naturally. If you meet a lot of women in bars, then every woman you meet will probably have dilated pupils, so don't take this sign too seriously. You also never know who's wearing contacts and how that may affect her eyes. Nonetheless, I have on occasion noticed that when I have complimented a woman, her pupils immediately expanded for a second or two. I can only assume that this is her natural response to my compliment.

3. Smile and Show Enthusiasm

This may seem like a no-brainer, but given the tendency of so many men to mislead women with their body language, it's worth repeating: You've got to smile and show enthusiasm if you want to convey interest in a conversation (and a person!). Simply put, a smile just opens people up, makes them feel more relaxed, and encourages them to talk to you and share things with you.

In my day-to-day interactions, I've noticed that most people have a fairly unpleasant look on their face throughout the course of the day. Most people don't purposely wear a grimace; that's just their natural expression when they don't pay any attention to it. It's sad that most people's normal expressions look more like frowns than they do smiles.

When someone does occasionally smile at me, I always notice because it occurs so rarely. Let's face it, most people are too busy to even look up, make eye contact, and smile at a passing stranger. So when someone does smile at me, I take notice and think to myself, "Wow, what a great person. I can't believe she took the time to smile at me." I've also realized that if a smile makes me feel that great, then imagine how great it must make others feel. I try to always walk around with a smile on my face. Yes, this is difficult, and I don't always succeed at it. However, when I'm walking down the street or when I enter an elevator, I glance around and smile at the people around me.

Ever since I started making an effort to smile, I've noticed that other people smile back at me more often. It sounds corny, but it's almost as if smiles are contagious. Regardless, if you don't want to make the effort to smile more in your daily life, at least make sure you smile when you're having a conversation with someone.

Enthusiasm goes hand in hand with smiling. Not only will you find it easier to smile when you're enthusiastic, but I've also found that when I smile, I'm naturally in a more upbeat mood. In *Make Every Girl Want You*™, Steve and I talked about the importance of enthusiasm and projecting the proper attitude. By smiling and projecting the proper (positive) attitude, you convey to someone that you're enjoying talking to her. I've seen a lot of guys do the exact opposite in conversations with women and fail miserably. What exactly is it that these guys – and maybe even you! – are doing wrong? Often, I see guys complaining to women they've just met, and I'm sorry to report that I've actually witnessed guys approach women with the following comments:

> "Oh, I can't believe how smoky it is in here!"

> "Why is this place always so loud?"

> "It's so hot in here; I wish I hadn't worn this sweater. But it's so cold outside that I would have been freezing on the way over here."

Although these statements seem relatively benign, they're actually complaints. I have yet to meet a woman who told me that she wants to be with a guy who's a complainer. When you initiate a conversation by complaining like these guys did, you've already got one strike against you. I've also seen guys complain about their jobs or their ex-girlfriends in their initial conversation with a woman. Attractive? Most women think not. While it's OK to share your problems with a woman when you're in a relationship, my friend Olivia relates that it's such a disappointment – and even kind of infuriating – to meet a guy who's a whiner:

"Oh, I met the most annoying guy last night. He started talking to me in the bathroom line, which was good timing because I was standing there by myself. But the first thing he said to me was, 'Seriously, could this bathroom line be any longer? You'd think a bar as popular as this one could afford to build some extra stalls or something.' I thought to myself, 'OK, no big deal.' I was actually flattered that he wanted to talk to me, so I dismissed that first complaint as a necessary opening line. But next thing I knew, he was complaining about his job and this city.

He went on and on about how he only moved to Boise for his job and how much he misses Chicago. I was offended from the beginning. I mean, I chose to move to this city, and I don't like it when anyone – much less a guy I've just met – badmouths Boise. This is my home, and I felt like he was telling me, 'You've got terrible taste. I can't believe you'd ever choose to live in a place like this.'

It only went downhill from there. Luckily, I made it to the bathroom relatively soon after that, but then he found me and my friends later in the evening and told us a really offensive joke. Why do I always meet such losers?"

It should be evident, then, that enthusiasm counts for a lot, particularly when you're first getting to know someone. Smiling and showing a little enthusiasm can't be that hard, particularly when the alternative means getting rejected by every woman you talk – or rather, complain – to.

4. Open Up Your Body Language

Unfold your arms, uncross your legs, and face the woman whom you're talking to with open body language. Learn to relax your body. I've seen some guys approach women and stand there stiff as a board. Of course, as with the earlier discussion about dilating pupils, you shouldn't get too caught up in trying to interpret someone else's body language. Just because a woman is standing there with her arms crossed doesn't mean that she doesn't want to talk to you. She may be cold, or that may be how she always stands.

In one of my recent courses, someone asked me if I agreed with "mirroring." I had never heard of this concept at that point, but I consulted my friend Kaitlyn, a sociologist who confirmed that mirroring does in fact work. When mirroring, you mimic the other person's body motions during a conversation as if you are the person's reflection in a mirror. For example, if a woman leans forward and rests her head on her right hand, you would lean forward and rest your head on your left hand. Similarly, if a woman steps forward a little bit with her left foot, you would step forward a little bit with your right foot.

Apparently, according to Kaitlyn, when you mirror someone's body motions, you begin to establish a connection with that person. Kaitlyn even mentioned that this is a popular technique that salesmen often use when talking to a customer. In fact, she said this often works so well that the salesman will take the lead and create a shift in his body motion, noticing that the customer follows his body movements without even realizing it! Listen to Kaitlyn's account of a friend of hers named Jake:

> "My friend Jake who's a salesman is so good at mirroring that after he starts mirroring his customers and then gets them to start mirroring him, he will ask a

question or push the product while nodding his head. He's told me that his customers will often nod in agreement without even realizing it."

Of course, when you mirror someone, don't make it obvious that you're mirroring her. When you first start mirroring someone, it's OK to wait a few moments until after she moves before mirroring her body movements. Over time, the two of you will get in sync to the point where you can make a movement, and the person will mimic you almost immediately.

Personally, I've never used mirroring or observed it in action. However, now that I'm aware of it, I'm sure I'll start to notice other people using it. Personally, I think those who mirror tote a fine line between being honest and messing with someone's head, and as a professional Nice Guy™, I prefer to avoid techniques that mess with a person's subconscious. Nonetheless, I included this subject in this book in hopes of leaving no question unanswered.

5. Nod Your Head

Nodding is an important part of the communication process that you probably never even think about. But if those plastic bobble heads can do it, you should definitely be able to nod as well if you put your mind – and head – to it. There are three types of nods, all of which send a different signal to the speaker. A single nod indicates that you agree with what the person is saying or that you're responding affirmatively to a question. Multiple nods, executed slowly and methodically, are used to convey that you understand what the person is saying as he or she offers up a drawn-out explanation. For example, just now at the gas station, I watched the clerk give a man directions. Their interaction went something like this:

Clerk: "Go back down the turnpike, until it

hooks up with the highway."
Man nodded: "OK"
Clerk: "Get back on the interstate headed east
for three miles."
Man nodded: "OK"
Clerk: "Take exit 74B, Route 1 South."
Man nodded: "OK"
Clerk: "Go up two traffic lights on Route 1."
Man nodded: "OK"
Clerk: "And you'll see it right there on your left.
You can't miss it."
Man nodded: "Oh, OK"
Man nodded: "Thank you."

You've probably also had plenty of interactions like this one. In this situation, you'll notice that there's often no need to actually speak. Nodding frequently does the trick.

A third type of nod, on the other hand, signals that the nodding person needs to say something. If you've ever nodded frequently and rapidly while another person is speaking, then you know exactly what I'm talking about. This frequent, rapid nod sends the signal that the listener has something to say. By nodding rapidly, it's almost as if the listener is trying to rush the speaker through his or her story so that he or she can then speak.

One of the most frustrating things when you have something to say is when someone else won't stop talking. Think about it: When someone else is talking, and it suddenly reminds you of something that you want to share, you sit there anxiously waiting for the other person to finish up so that you can interject. When a woman sends you that signal that she wants to say something, quickly finish up what you have to say and cede the floor to her. Remember, most people would rather talk than listen, so if a woman's got something to say, let her speak. You don't want to become known as the guy who thinks the world revolves around him. Besides, you can always fill in the gaps of silence later by resuming your story.

While these three types of nods send various signals, a lack of nodding sends a signal that you're simply not interested in what the person has to say. Be conscious of yourself if you tend not to nod when listening to someone else. It is a natural human reaction to nod during conversation, and you probably do it without even thinking. However, I've observed some people who just don't nod during a conversation. It's a shame because they're conveying indifference when that probably isn't their intention. If you're one of these people who needs to integrate nodding into your repertoire of conversational techniques, then it's most important that you start using the second nod I discussed: the slow, methodical nod that conveys interest in a conversation.

Much like the aforementioned man and clerk at the gas station, Oscar nods in conversation every time either he or his conversational partner makes a point. I've observed Oscar and, on average, the nods seem to occur at a rate of one every two-and-a-half to three seconds. Of course, the exact frequency of nods depends upon the speed of the conversation. In conversations with a faster speed, Oscar nods more frequently. In slower conversations, there is a longer lapse between head nods. If you're one of these people who doesn't naturally nod in conversation, the variation in nod frequency may sound complicated. However, it is likely to come naturally to you, as it does for Oscar, if you just start paying attention to your body language and making an effort to nod. One of my friends, Katelyn, recently told me about a guy she knows who never nods in conversation:

> "It's really weird. Christian doesn't really know how to show that he's listening during a conversation. I mean, he makes good eye contact, but it's kind of like he's in a trance. He doesn't bother to nod, or

say 'uh-huh' every few seconds, like most people do. So I really don't feel like he's listening to me."

6. Maintain an Appropriate Distance

While I was on the train a couple of weeks ago, I struck up a conversation with the woman sitting across from me. This was a typical passenger train with an aisle in the middle and two seats on either side. Because she and I were sitting on the opposite sides of the aisle from each other in our respective window seats, we were seated the furthest possible distance apart from each other.

A little bored and always looking to meet new women, I struck up a conversation with her. Although I started with some small talk, we were fully engaged in conversation after about a minute and a half. At that point, she slid over into the aisle seat with her arm resting on the armrest closest to the aisle in order to move closer to me, so I too slid over to my aisle seat to better engage in the conversation.

Notice that even as we slid toward each other, we still maintained a distance of two to three feet because the aisle stood between us. It would have been rude for her to cross the aisle and sit on my side of the aisle because, as a stranger, she would then be invading my space. Likewise, she probably would have felt that I was violating her space if I had suddenly gotten up and sat in the seat next to her less than three minutes after meeting her.

Everyone has what's known as his or her own "personal space," which is typically about two feet in front of you. No one really likes to be any closer than two feet from someone whom they've just met. Any closer than this would be considered an invasion of that person's space, and some women may even interpret this in a threatening manner.

Most people naturally understand everyone's need for his or her own space, but some people seem to have never picked up on this. I've seen many guys approach women and stand within a foot or even six inches of her face during their very first meeting, as if he was about to lean in and kiss her. In each instance, this made the woman feel very uncomfortable, and the woman continually backed away. In many cases, this caused the guy to lose confidence since he didn't understand why the woman was retreating. He hadn't said anything wrong; he was merely invading her space.

While violating someone's personal space can be a turn-off, particularly during an initial meeting, testing someone's space is a good way to see how close a person feels to you after a certain point. I've noticed that when I'm out on a successful date, the woman will often gradually move closer to me throughout the evening to the point where we're often, for instance, standing on a boardwalk chatting no more than six inches from each other's face. When a woman willingly engages in a conversation with you on a date, while standing only six inches from your face, this means that she feels extremely comfortable around you and most likely wants you to kiss her.

Conversely, keep in mind that sometimes a woman's distance from you may have nothing to do with you at all. When you're not feeling well, your desire to have your own space increases. If you have a headache, you want to be left alone and don't want anyone within ten feet of you. Likewise, a woman with whom you may have been very intimate three days ago may not want to sit right next to you on the couch while watching a movie today. Yes, this could mean that she no longer wants to be intimate with you, but it could also mean that she simply isn't feeling well and doesn't feel like sharing her space right now. You shouldn't suddenly jump the gun and assume that things are off just because she needs a little space of her own.

Finally, it's important to realize that the importance of personal space varies from culture to culture. I've noticed that in some other countries, people tend to stand much closer to each other when they're having a conversation. Sometimes this causes a problem as people immigrate to America from other countries and don't realize that they're violating the space of others. Guys who have come to the U.S. from foreign countries in which personal space is kept to a minimum and being touchy-feely is acceptable often walk up to women, stand very close to them, and touch them a lot during the initial conversation. By witnessing such interactions, I have learned that this violation of personal space, particularly by a stranger, often makes women feel very uncomfortable. My friend Jessica said the following about Rick, a guy from another country who tends to stand too close during conversations:

> "What is it with Rick? Whenever I talk to him, he hovers over me like he's about to lean in and kiss me. I mean, he's the nicest guy on the planet. He's always really friendly, but he just has no concept of personal space. Whenever we're talking, I find myself repeatedly backing away. But that just seems to draw him in closer.
>
> The scariest was the other day at work when I ended up backing all the way up to a wall. There I was, standing with my back to a wall, and Rick was still six inches from my face. Finally, I just had to pretend that I was late to a meeting to get away from him."

The funny thing is that Rick also confided in me:

> "John, I don't know what the problem is. Whenever I talk to women, they back away from me. I mean, I thought maybe I smelled bad or had bad breath or something. So I started showering twice a day, and now I always make it a point to

shower before I go out. I always brush my teeth after every meal and before going out at night. I've even started chewing gum a lot. I use extra cologne. I just can't figure it out. Do I smell that bad? Is it my breath? What is it??"

I, of course, explained to Rick what the problem was. At first he was shocked, and then he was just embarrassed. He corrected the problem immediately, and there hasn't been another incident since then. Rick and I can laugh about it since his confidence has drastically increased now that women no longer back away when he approaches them. Rick, I'm proud to say, has become a successful Nice Guy.

7. Confidently Shake Hands

I often get asked about when it is appropriate to touch someone. For starters, the only physical contact you should have with someone whom you have just met or barely know is a handshake.

When Oscar walks into a room full of people that he knows, he makes sure to go around and shake everyone's hand. For instance, I remember once when a bunch of guys got together to watch a football game a couple of years ago, Oscar was the last one there. However, when he arrived, he walked up to each guy in the room one-by-one, confidently extending his arm, looking the guy in the eyes, and saying one of the following:

"Hey, <name>. Good to see you."
"Hey, <name>. How've you been?"

Similarly, I've noticed that whenever Oscar sees a woman whom he knows, he always goes up and hugs her. Not surprisingly, the woman always reciprocates. I've always noticed, however, that if it's a woman whom Oscar is meeting for the first time or has met once or twice before but doesn't know very well, then he'll respect her space and extend a confident handshake instead. While it's impressive that Oscar shakes hands with women he barely knows, the real reason that this guy is the poster child for The Nice Guys™ is that he always walks up and initiates the conversation when there are people in the room whom he doesn't know – regardless of whether they're men or women. For example, when we were watching that football game, there were two guys visiting one of our friends from out of town. After Oscar had greeted everyone else in the room, he immediately went up to the two guys he didn't know, extended his arm for a handshake, and introduced himself.

This friendly behavior of the quintessential Nice Guy has an amazing side effect, which I first discovered while observing Oscar and later found to be true based on firsthand experience. When you make it a point to walk up to and naturally and confidently introduce yourself to strangers at a party or social gathering, it will only be natural for you to do the same with attractive women. Back in my pathetic days, I used to be *extremely* insecure about introducing myself to beautiful women. Their beauty was so intimidating that I acted as if they were superhuman rather than normal human beings like you and me. These days I don't even think twice about introducing myself to attractive women. In a room full of people, I introduce myself, one-by-one, to each person throughout the course of the evening. By not differentiating between anyone in the room, I'm sure to meet all of the beautiful women with no added pressure.

I guess you could say I figured this out the hard way a few years ago when I went out with Oscar to a wine tasting party at a mutual friend's apartment. Both of us knew Ashley, the hostess, but neither of us knew many other people there. At one point in the evening, Ashley introduced us to four friends of hers. I merely held up my hand, waved hello, and said, "Hey, I'm John." Oscar took the time to individually shake each woman's hand and introduce himself, looking each woman in the eye in the process. Oscar confidently repeated each woman's name back to her while shaking her hand, such as, "Hi, Beth, I'm Oscar, very nice to meet you." Fifteen minutes later, these women were drooling over Oscar, and I was merely a mannequin standing next to him. I have since learned to never mass-introduce myself to people, and now I always take the time to personally introduce myself to everyone one-by-one. This conveys the message, "I'm interested in you as a person," which has the effect of making the person in question feel important. My good friend Ashley relays her first impression of Oscar:

> "I'll never forget when I first met Oscar; it was at Megan's birthday party. Megan introduced him to me, and Oscar firmly shook my hand, looked me in the eyes, and said, 'Ashley, it's really nice to meet you.' No guy has ever done that to me before! I knew right then that this guy was special!"

Here's a final word of advice about handshakes: I've found from watching Oscar and other really confident guys that it's not just about the quantity of handshakes; it's also about the *quality* of the handshakes. In a good handshake, your hands meet so that the fleshy piece of skin between your thumb and your first finger touch. You then firmly squeeze the person's hand for a second or two and release. This sends an unmistakable signal of confidence to men and women alike. One of the worst mistakes in handshaking – and I'm surprised how many guys make this mistake – is squeezing someone's fingers. If you don't extend your hand far enough and prematurely squeeze, then you'll end up squeezing the person's fingers together, which can be especially painful if he or she is wearing a ring. Jamming the person's ring down into his or her finger is just about the last thing you want to do when you're meeting someone for the first time, regardless of whether the person in question is an executive at work or a beautiful and potentially dateable woman. Not only is it embarrassing, but it also exposes your apprehension and suggests that your social skills are lacking.

8. Match Speed and Volume

Have you ever found yourself in a situation where you were incredibly excited about something, but the woman you were seeing was quite distraught over something else? In a world full of independent women, it's not unusual to find yourself in a drastically different emotional state than your girlfriend or wife. How do you have a conversation with her in these situations? Steve and I began answering this question in *Make Every Girl Want You*™ when we discussed emotion matching. We advise that if the woman is happy during conversation, act happy with her. Similarly, if she is sad or upset, respond in a mellow tone. Oscar is the king of emotion matching. If a woman is jovial, upbeat, laughing, or happy, Oscar will respond in the same manner. If a woman is upset or bothered, Oscar takes on a very serious look.

For emotion matching to be effective, it's important to try to match your conversational partner's speed and volume. For instance, I've noticed that Oscar doesn't simply mimic his conversational partner's emotions; he also matches her speed and volume. If she is speaking slowly and quietly, he will respond slowly and quietly. If she is excited and relaying a story very rapidly and animatedly, he accelerates his rate of speaking.

Unfortunately for them, I've seen plenty of guys do the exact opposite by counteracting the emotion of the woman they're talking to. I've watched other guys who respond a mile a minute while talking to a woman who's speaking slowly and quietly. This has a tendency to completely overwhelm the woman. If you do this, you'll make a woman feel uncomfortable and discourage her from having future conversations with you – or worse yet, from dating you.

Some men naturally speak with loud, booming voices, which can be very intimidating to women. These men typically speak loudly not because they can't speak softly, but rather they do so as a matter of expression. If you're one such guy, learn to speak a little more softly and project less when you're in a one-on-one conversation with someone so you don't overwhelm her and scare her away.

When you're engaged in a conversation with a woman, she wants to feel like you're speaking directly to her. If you speak softly and look her in the eyes, as Oscar always does, you effectively convey that you are talking solely to her. When you speak with a loud, booming voice, on the other hand, it's as if you're trying to advertise your conversation and want to be overheard by everyone around you. This sends a message to the woman that you don't really care about having a conversation with her as much as you're just speaking to turn a few heads.

I've actually noticed some guys who purposely speak loudly, hoping that other women will overhear them and get involved in the conversation. This strategy usually backfires since it both sends a negative message to the woman with whom they're talking and sends a message to the surrounding women that this guy is loud, obnoxious, and not worth speaking to. As my friend Anna remarked:

> "I hate guys who are loud talkers. I have such a soft voice, and those guys just overwhelm me. It's also a big turn-off when I hear a guy with a booming voice because I feel like he doesn't just want to talk to me. It seems like he just wants attention; he wants everyone around to hear him. When I'm talking to a guy, I want to know that he's interested in

having a conversation with me and isn't talking loudly enough for the entire room to hear."

Notice that Anna doesn't criticize a guy's tone of voice here. She's not saying that if you have a deep voice, you should start speaking as if you've been castrated. But if a woman's word is any indication (and I assume it is since you're reading this book!), changing the speed and volume at which you speak to match that of your conversational partner's can go a long way in maintaining a woman's interest.

9. Don't over-interpret someone else's body language

The reason that I wrote this chapter was to encourage you to pay more attention to yourself and the manner in which you convey – or fail to convey – interest in a conversation. However, you shouldn't necessarily assume that a woman isn't interested in what you have to say just because she isn't making eye contact with you or because she's standing there with her arms crossed. It's entirely possible that she was just never taught how to convey interest in a conversation. The bottom line is that you shouldn't make too many assumptions about someone else's body language. I have quite a few female friends who over-interpret body language. Here are three examples in which verbal communication would have gone a long way:

> Samantha: "Yeah, I know Lauren doesn't like me. Did you see the way she walked by and wouldn't even look at me?"

Because of this, Samantha started behaving unpleasantly toward Lauren. When Lauren then observed how Samantha was behaving, she refused to speak to Samantha. They didn't speak for a week.

> Megan: "I walked up to her and I said, 'Hi, Grace.' She said 'hi' back, but she wasn't smiling at all. I guess she is still mad at me."

Because of this, Megan started ignoring Grace. When Grace realized this, she complained to me,

> "Wow, Megan's being really pissy toward me."

They didn't speak for two weeks.

> Alana: "Whenever I walk by, Gabrielle looks at me as if I'm not good enough to be here. I'm not speaking to her anymore."

Because of this, Alana refused to talk to Gabrielle. Gabrielle came up and asked me,

> "Um, John, is Alana upset with me? Did I do something wrong?"

They ended up not speaking for two weeks.

In all three cases, two of my female friends ended up not speaking to each other for at least a week simply because one friend overanalyzed the other friend's body language. Let's look back at what was actually going on in each of these instances:

> Lauren's mom was in the hospital, and thus her body language was negative toward everyone that evening.

> Grace had just had a root canal, so she couldn't smile at anyone.

Gabrielle was allergic to Alana's perfume, and that's why she winced every time Alana walked by.

While it's important to pay attention to body language, make sure you don't prematurely draw negative conclusions from body language. Each of these situations would have been resolved much more easily – and quickly – if the woman who overanalyzed the other's body language had simply pulled the person aside and asked her:

"Hey, are you upset with me?"

"I noticed you walked by earlier and didn't even say hi. Are you still mad at me?"

"Hey, I noticed we haven't been talking much lately. Is everything OK with you? Did I do something that offended you?"

Yes, it really could've been that simple for my friends to resolve their problems. But at least you now know what to do if you ever let your imagination run wild and jump to conclusions too quickly when you try to read people's body language.

So now that you know the do's and don'ts of conveying interest in a conversation, the next step is to keep the conversation going long enough to get a woman's contact info! Read on, as the next chapter will provide advice on keeping your conversations flowing smoothly.

Chapter 6 – The Nice Guys' Guide™ to Not Talking about Yourself

Steve and I, in *Make Every Girl Want You*™, stressed the importance of not talking about yourself. But despite our valiant effort, it appears that most guys just don't get it, which does not bode well for our gender. As I've learned, talking about oneself nonstop is the single largest error that most guys make. Whenever women find out that I'm an author and speaker on the topic of meeting women, they always ask, "So, what's the #1 thing that you tell guys?" As I tell them – and now you – the single most important piece of advice for guys is this: When you first meet a woman, don't try to impress her by talking about yourself!

You should see women's reactions when I tell them this. They always unanimously nod in agreement and then start telling me their stories of every guy – just today! – who has approached them and talked about himself nonstop. Guys, at the risk of saying something that the Nike advertising department would most definitely consider sacrilegious, I beg you: *Just don't do it.* Don't talk about yourself. You might think that the way to impress a woman is by talking about yourself, but unfortunately: You're wrong. The quickest way to turn a woman off is to talk about yourself.

There were at least three men at a wedding that I went to last Saturday who learned that the hard way. I spoke with three different women of varying ages about this problem, and all three concurred with me. A sixteen-year-old named Elizabeth complained:

> "Oh, my gosh! You're so right. There's actually this guy who won't leave me alone today. He's following me around; he keeps trying to talk to me. All he does is talk nonstop about his wrestling team and about how he's the #1 wrestler on the team and how he might win the state championship this year. Ugh! Just leave me alone!"

Audrey, a twenty-four-year-old woman whom I met at the wedding, rolled her eyes and said:

> "I couldn't tell you how much I agree. The guy who sat next to me during dinner was a lawyer, and all he talked about was himself. How he's the world's greatest lawyer, about how he breezed through law school, about all the cases he's won. Ugh! If I hear one more word about being a lawyer . . .
>
> And the sad thing is that he's not a bad-looking guy. He just has no clue how to have a conversation with a woman. If he would just shut up about himself, I might try to take him home with me tonight!"

Judy, a thirty-five-year-old woman whom I met, had had a similar conversation:

> "Yeah, that guy who I was dancing with earlier – what a great dancer! I had so much fun dancing with him! Unfortunately, the fun ended abruptly when we stopped dancing and he opened his mouth. He wouldn't shut up about his boat and his two homes.
>
> He just went on and on about his 35-foot yacht that he keeps parked at the marina and takes out on the weekends, and his home up in New York and his home down in Florida. Blah blah blah. Did he honestly think he was impressing me with that? Seriously! I was so turned off by it that I have no desire to dance with him again even though he's a great dancer!"

Hopefully, these conversations illustrate that this problem isn't unique to one type of guy. It doesn't matter whether you're a seventeen-year-old wrestler or a fifty-two-year-old man with a boat and two homes. Whatever your age and interests, there's a good chance that you have this problem of talking about yourself more than any woman can bear to listen to. It doesn't matter what age the woman is. She could be in high school or in her fifties. It really doesn't make a difference. No woman wants to hear you talk about yourself nonstop.

Even after all of this, I wouldn't be surprised if you're thinking, "I can't help it. It's just easier for me to talk about myself since that's what I know the most about." You can pull this off, trust me. Oscar does it all the time. You will rarely hear Oscar talk about himself. When he does, it's only a little bit at a time, and it's only after asking a woman a question about herself first. Women are so attracted to Oscar precisely because he expresses genuine interest in others before talking about himself. Go ahead, try it. You just might surprise yourself. Who knows, you might even surprise a few women!

Reticence

I often hear the following:

> "You've mentioned reticence and advised guys to be reticent when first meeting women. Can you please expand on that? What exactly should we avoid discussing the first time we meet a woman?"

As Steve and I said in *Make Every Girl Want You*™, reticence simply means keeping your strongest opinions to yourself initially. I'm not saying that you shouldn't express yourself, but use a little discretion the first time you're meeting someone, be it a man or a woman. We at The Nice Guys' Institute™ consider the following topics taboo during an introductory conversation:

- Tragedies, adversities, or misfortunes, particularly recent occurrences. For example, you probably shouldn't say, "Yeah, I lost my dad ten years ago. Has anyone else here lost their dad?" You never know when someone's dad may currently be in poor health or may have recently passed away. The only exception to this is when the other person brought it up first. In which case, you should proceed with caution.
- Health in general. Don't rattle off your medical history or your current ailments, and don't pry about someone else's health concerns. This is personal stuff that most

people don't want to discuss, particularly with someone they just met. The only exception to this rule is if you meet someone on crutches (or someone with a broken arm). In this case, the person's health condition isn't fatal and is apparent even to a total stranger, which makes mentioning it an easy and appropriate icebreaker: "I'm sorry about your foot. Can I ask what happened?" Here you can simultaneously offer up compassion and keep the conversation going for a little while longer.

- Conversations about money, particularly expensive purchases. For instance, never ask how much someone paid for her car. It's poor form, and it makes you look like you're obsessed with money. If the guy with the two homes and a yacht was any indication, talking about money or possessions is likely to turn women off.

- Any story that could be considered tasteless or offensive. Remember, women are more likely to consider a story tasteless or offensive than men are, so you shouldn't necessarily speak to a woman the same way that you talk to your male friends when you're watching football or checking out women. Always use caution when telling a story. If you're not quite sure what should be off-limits, we provide some examples of what *not* to say in *Make Every Girl Want You*™.

- Any controversial topic, such as abortion, gun control, or the death penalty. People tend to have very emotional stances on these issues, and it is best to avoid them in an introductory conversation. Remember, you don't get a second chance to make a first impression.

- Views on others' lifestyles. If you don't like others who are different from you, whether it's because they are of a different religion, nationality, or sexual preference, that is none of my business. However, do NOT even think about voicing this opinion in an introductory conversation with others. I have witnessed guys who had been charming a beautiful woman up until that point shoot themselves in the foot by making a joke about homosexuality, not realizing that her brother is gay. Regardless of whether you think the joke is funny, you never know whose sister, brother, father, or mother is gay, has Down Syndrome, or is from a foreign country. What you do behind closed doors is certainly none of my business. Sure, there's a chance that she may find your impersonation of a kid with Down Syndrome funny. But if you make fun of a kid with Down Syndrome and her brother has the disease (or anyone who overheard you has a relative or friend with that disease), it will take years for you to earn back her respect.

- Politics and religion – both best saved for future discussions.

Although, in this book, we attempted to present a lot of material on approaching women, there is still a lot more that even we at *The Nice Guys' Institute*™ have yet to discover. We get asked more questions about approaching women than anything else, and are currently compiling a report of the most frequently-asked questions. When we are finished, we will either post the report on www.TheNiceGuysGuide.com, or include it in a future book.

Visit the site often as we are constantly updating it with new content, including downloadable e-books and e-reports, audio tapes and CDs, and video cassettes and DVDs packed with our latest discoveries. We also maintain information on our web site about upcoming coaching sessions, course offerings, and speaking engagements. Additionally, we encourage readers to e-mail us, either through our web site, or at TheNiceGuys@TheNiceGuysGuide.com. Finally, please also come by and sign up for our free newsletter to receive the hottest tips to help nice guys like you make themselves more attractive to women WITHOUT turning into jerks!

Part III The Nice Guys' Guide™ to the Movies, Oral Sex, Getting Your Ex Back, and Friendships with Women

In Part III of The Nice Guys' Guide™, I will offer further advice on a range of topics that didn't fit neatly into any other section. This includes:

In the "From Dating to a Relationship" chapter of Make Every Girl Want You™, Steve and I discussed the importance of selflessly performing oral sex on a woman the first time you are intimate with her. In Part III of The Nice Guys' Guide™, we at The Nice Guys' Institute™ seek to answer the hundreds of questions from guys who have e-mailed us asking for advice on this matter by offering tips on performing top-notch oral sex that will leave your woman begging for more (and telling all of her friends)!

Additionally, we at The Nice Guys' Institute™ often get asked what the best approach is for winning back your ex. In Part III of The Nice Guys' Guide™, we will offer advice on this topic.

Chapter 7 – The Nice Guys' Guide™ to Performing Oral Sex

I had such a great time last night. I ended up hanging out with a few good female friends of mine – none of whom I'm hooking-up with, I'll have you know. It was raining, so we stayed in and opened a couple of bottles of Chianti.

I think we were on our third or fourth glass of Chianti when the conversation suddenly turned to oral sex. The discussion that ensued for the next hour and a half was incredible not only because I was surrounded by a bunch of beautiful women talking about oral sex but also because of what I learned from our conversation. Even after all that wine, I couldn't wait to get up first thing this morning and write a chapter about it.

In the "From Dating to a Relationship" chapter of *Make Every Girl Want You*™, Steve and I made note of the importance of performing good oral sex on a woman. For those of you who missed it the first time, let me reiterate: When you get the chance to perform oral sex on a woman for the first time, do so. Go down on her for a long time. Give her orgasm after orgasm, and don't worry about yourself. Don't focus on whether or not she has returned the favor. Focus only on pleasuring her. Continue making her cum, spend the night with her, and perform oral sex on her again in the morning.

Why would you want to be so selfless? Well, let's just say that women love well-performed oral sex. My conversation with my friends last night definitely confirmed this. Many women find it difficult to have an orgasm from intercourse, especially the first few times with a new partner. Almost every woman, however, can have an orgasm from properly performed oral sex. As we said in *Make Every Girl Want You*™, if you are successful, she'll not only want you in her bed every night – and day! – of the year, but she'll also tell all of her friends just how good you are! My friend Denise said it all:

> "When I find that rare guy who is actually good at oral sex, he's welcome in my bed any night of the year! He's the guy who's going on my speed dial and who's likely to get a drunk dial from me every Friday night around 2 AM!"

After she said that, the roomful of women broke into a round of applause. I guess we know how women feel about well-performed oral sex! You should have heard these girls squeal simply by recalling the best orgasms they've received from oral sex. All I can say is that if their recollections were that good, those guys must've done something right! That being said, I'm now going to relay to you exactly how women like oral sex performed on them.

The first rule that I learned from these women is to never go straight down on a woman. According to my female friends, some of the most inexperienced guys they've been with thought that oral sex was a mechanism purely for arousing a woman for intercourse. They all agreed that many inexperienced guys went straight down on them before they were even aroused, played around briefly, and then came back up and wanted to engage in intercourse. For the women, these guys left much to be desired in bed.

According to my friends, guys who know what they're doing first spend the time to get them aroused by kissing, stroking, and licking the rest of their body, and then move on to oral sex once the woman is sufficiently aroused. So, the first rule is to take the time to kiss, lick, and stroke the woman all over – on her lips, face, neck, shoulders, breasts, nipples, arms, fingers, stomach, thighs, calves, and even in between her breasts – before performing oral sex. When done slowly and intimately, this foreplay will sufficiently arouse a woman to want to receive oral sex and subsequently engage in intercourse.

When you do go down on a woman to perform oral sex, start by gently stroking and licking her inner thighs rather than licking her vagina right away. Spending a few moments on a woman's thighs as you slowly approach her vagina can really arouse her as she builds up anticipation about what's next on the agenda.

Before you go any further, it's useful to be familiar with the female anatomy, particularly if you want to be the guy that ends up on her speed dial. For those of you who weren't biology majors (don't worry, neither was I), here's a quick anatomy lesson: When you look at a woman's vulva (the vaginal area), you will see a pair of lips. They look more or less like the lips you'd see on someone's face, except that they're turned vertically. There are actually two pairs of lips, the outer lips (called the *labia majoris*) and the inner lips (called the *labia minoris*). Depending on the position you are viewing a woman from and how aroused she is at the moment, you may or may not see the inner lips.

At the top of the lips is a little mound known as the clitoris. The clitoris, when un-aroused, has a hood over it. As a woman becomes aroused, the clitoris will often (but not always) peak out from under its hood. You can recognize it as a little pink bud peering out. In some women, however, their clitoris remains hidden behind its hood even when they are at their highest point of arousal.

The clitoris is the central point of stimulation for a woman, much like the head of a man's penis is for a man. You can stroke a man's penis all day long, but unless you pay attention to the head, it's very difficult to cum. Likewise, you can lick a woman's labia all day long, but unless you eventually work your way toward the clitoris, it is very difficult to make a woman cum. There is an important distinction, however. A woman can start licking the head of a man's penis the second he gets an erection, and it will lead to orgasm. A man, on the other hand, should never go straight for a woman's clitoris. As we're about to discuss, you should spend some time on the labia first.

A word of caution: most women have told me that their clitoris is *extremely* sensitive. Unlike with the head of a penis, in which you want a woman to apply direct sensation with her tongue, most women have said that direct sensation is often too much, and it may hurt. My female friends suggest that a guy should merely flick at the clitoris with his tongue or suck on the hood surrounding the clitoris (but not the clitoris itself). One of my friends, Gabby, talks about a very painful experience:

> "Oh, man. This guy, well, I really shouldn't say his name. But he had no clue what he was doing. I've heard guys talk about painful oral sex – girls who scraped them, but man this particular *guy* had to be worse than any woman who's bad at oral sex.
>
> So he went down on me, and put my entire clitoris in his mouth. The entire clitoris – hood and all – in his mouth and

starting humming! It hurt like hell! I'm guessing that's what he wants me to do to him: take him entirely in my mouth and hum. But *please* don't ever do that to a woman, unless she specifically asks! This guy was obviously an amateur when it comes to oral sex. He obviously doesn't know much about a woman's body! We're way too sensitive for that maneuver!"

So where do we start? Commence oral sex by slowly licking a woman's outer lips up and down with your tongue without actually inserting your tongue. After doing this for a little bit, part her outer lips with your tongue (not your fingers!). Work your way through to her inner lips and slowly lick them up and down. If you can't work your way through to her inner lips with your tongue alone, it is OK to use your hands to help pull her outer lips apart. The more you do with your tongue, however, the better it will feel to her.

Next, move your tongue inside her vagina. Apparently this is where many guys start – they just part the woman's lips open and start moving their tongue in and out. Women prefer the technique that I mentioned: taking your time and slowly lick her lips first. Once your tongue is inside her vagina, move it in and out and up and down. Listen to her cues. If she moans a lot when you use a particular tongue motion, then keep doing it (more on oral cues in a moment).

Realize, however, that moving your tongue around her vagina isn't the endpoint. According to my female friends, a lot of guys just move their tongues in and out of their vaginas or move their tongue up and down on their lips. Meanwhile, they're missing the whole point of performing oral sex on a woman: the clitoris!

Once the woman is sufficiently lubricating from everything you've done so far, move on to her clitoris. As mentioned, this area is extremely sensitive, so proceed with caution. Start by licking the hood of the clitoris. Hopefully, her clitoris will be peering out at you like a little pink bud by this point. If that is the case, then flick at her clitoris with your tongue. Listen to her moans and responses, and go with whatever she appears to enjoy the most! Just keep in mind that her clitoris is very sensitive. Some women prefer that you put your lips around the hood of their clitoris and suck on it; for other women, the clitoris is much too sensitive for such a maneuver.

The most important advice I can give you about performing oral sex on a woman is to listen to her responses. Very few women will tell you, "OK. Put your lips around the hood of my clitoris and suck lightly." But most women are very adept at providing cues orally through their moans. No matter what you're doing, listen to a woman's moans. Remember that every woman is different. A particular tongue movement that worked great on one woman may not work at all on another. My friend Chloe shared the following anecdote about a guy who mistakenly believed that he was good at oral sex:

> "This guy Brad actually got mad at me during oral sex because his 'move' didn't work on me! It's like he didn't understand – 'Hello! Every woman is different.' But he just sat there and swore that this was his trademark move and that he could make me cum even though it didn't feel that good. All he had to do was try something else – learn a new 'move'! Oh well, he's no longer allowed in my bedroom. That's alright. I have Austin's magical tongue now!"

The best advice I have for you is to be flexible and listen to a woman's cues. If she starts moaning when you try something, then keep doing it! If she doesn't really respond, try something else. Just don't ever take a one-size-fits-all approach to performing oral sex.

A lot of guys tell me that they don't know what to do with their hands during oral sex. I've learned that it is important to let your hands wander. Stroke her thighs, move your hands up to her breasts, caress her nipples, stroke her arms. Let your arms glide all over her entire body, and have some fun while your tongue does the work. My friend Maureen had this to say about using your hands during oral sex:

> "My ex-boyfriend Craig, who I still sleep with, gives me the most intense orgasms I've ever felt. For starters, he's actually good at oral sex, unlike any other guy I've been with. He actually takes his time, and slowly brings me to an orgasm. And it usually takes me a while, but he's very patient, and doesn't stop until I cum.
>
> But it's not just that he knows what to do with his tongue; there are plenty of guys who think they know that. What makes Craig different is he knows what to do with his hands as well! While his tongue is busy at work, he's often stroking my thighs, playing with my breasts, caressing my nipples, holding my hand, or running his hands all over my body.
>
> It's so intense that when I cum, I have a full-body orgasm – I can feel it in my entire body! It's *amazing* – I've never felt anything like it before!"

Another move that women tell me works really well is to insert a finger or two into her vagina as the woman is becoming extremely aroused. Notice that this doesn't mean you should stop licking her clitoral area;

this merely provides her with additional stimulation. I've actually found that saving that for the woman's second orgasm works really well. I prefer to bring a woman to orgasm using only my tongue the first time. Then, after she's cum once, I'll insert a finger or two into her vagina while continuing to lick her labia and her clitoral area. In my experience, this often helps bring the woman to an even more intense second orgasm.

When you insert your fingers into a woman's vagina, try to find her G-spot. Most guys have heard about the infamous G-spot, but most guys don't have a clue where to find it. In fact, a lot of women have no idea where it is or if they even have one. To this day, no one's really sure if every woman has a G-spot. But apparently, quite a few do, so you might as well go for it.

I tried reading up on the G-spot to try to figure out where it is. It was rather difficult to understand the scientific text I found, so let me try to explain it in much simpler terms. When you insert a finger or two into a woman's vagina, turn your arm so your palm is facing up. Gently curl your fingers toward yourself, as if you're issuing a "come here" motion. As you do this, the tips of your fingers should rub against the front wall of the woman's vagina. According to experts, there is often a rough patch on the front wall of the vagina where your fingers will be rubbing. This is what they dub the G-spot. It is a tiny area, but women who report having a G-spot say that the sensations caused by stimulating this area are tremendous. The next time you are performing oral sex, insert a finger or two into the woman's vagina and see if you can find her G-spot. If you feel the rough patch, continue massaging it with your fingers and see how she reacts. Of course, don't forget to keep your tongue busy while you're doing this.

After reading this, you might think you're an expert on performing oral sex, but there's one more important thing to keep in mind: Every female friend of mine whom I have asked has agreed that the biggest mistake that men make during oral sex is not finishing the job. As I said earlier, most guys treat oral sex as a means to intercourse rather than as an experience that is enjoyable in and of itself. My female friends have all suggested that oral sex is merely a starting point and that when they cum through oral sex, they just get even more aroused to have intercourse.

Unfortunately, it appears that most guys think that the female body operates like ours do. As a guy, you know that if you cum through oral sex, then you're done for a while. Depending on your age, it could take from ten minutes to a few hours before you're fully recharged! With women, it's quite the opposite. Women can have multiple orgasms in rapid succession. When you make a woman cum through oral sex, you're merely getting her more turned on to want to continue on to intercourse.

A lot of women can't cum just from intercourse; they require the clitoral stimulation that comes from oral sex. Because of this, a lot of women have also told me that they can only have an orgasm from intercourse *after* they've already cum from oral sex. They expressed that when a guy uses oral sex merely to turn them on and doesn't finish the job, then they're left very unsatisfied because they simply can't cum from intercourse unless they cum from oral sex first.

Don't be afraid to go all the way when you perform oral sex! In fact, make her cum multiple times through oral sex. While you might suspect that this would prevent the woman from having intercourse with you since she will have already cum, the opposite is true. She'll be turned on and want to have sex with you even more. Additionally, if you're good at oral sex, she'll want you back in her bed every night of the year. If you're lucky, she might even extend the invitation randomly during the daytime!

While in a room full of women talking about sex, I knew I couldn't pass up the opportunity to ask the obvious question, "Does size matter?" Here are a couple of the better responses:

> Cindy: "No, especially not if he's good with his tongue!"

> Abby: "I was with this one guy. I'm not going to say his name, but his thing was especially small. I think he knew it, though. Instead of being embarrassed about it (like another guy I dated), I guess he realized that he should just overcompensate in other areas. And overcompensate he did! He moved up to Philly, but I still sleep with him whenever he's in town."

The great thing about oral sex is that once you're good at it and your woman enjoys letting you perform oral sex on her, you can perform it in a number of different positions. Sure, there is the standard position in which the woman lies flat on her back and you lay down in between her legs.

There are alternate positions, however, such as the woman sitting upright on the edge of the bed with her legs dangling over the edge, and you kneeling on the floor beneath her. In fact, why restrict this position to a bed? A woman can sit, for example, on the kitchen counter or on a laundry machine (whose added vibrations may provide additional stimulation for her) with her legs dangling over the edge while you kneel beneath her and bring her to a tremendous orgasm. Women have told me that they often find risqué situations like these highly erotic and exciting, particularly if there's a chance that you might get caught!

Another variation that you may want to try is having the woman sit on your face and gently wriggle back and forth. In this position, the woman can take control and sway her torso back and forth over your tongue. Many women have told me that they love the power they feel by sitting on a guy's face.

Another well-known variation is commonly called 69. In this position, the woman performs oral sex on you while you simultaneously perform oral sex on her. A word of warning: It is often difficult for a woman to reach orgasm through 69. Women often need to relax and concentrate on their orgasms in order to be able to cum. If they're busy performing oral sex on you, many women will find that they are unable to cum. If this is the case, be sure to always continue performing oral sex on her in a relaxing position after you have cum. She will only want to engage in 69 in the future if you have taken the time to help her reach orgasm as well.

Another variation on oral sex is that in which the woman stands up, and the man kneels between her legs. Again, a lot of women have told me that they like this sexually dominant position, in which they get to stand up while a guy submissively kneels before them and licks them.

A few words of warning about what not to do during oral sex: First of all, never blow into a woman's vagina. This very dangerous maneuver can cause an embolism in the woman's body. When you blow into a woman's vagina, an air bubble can travel up through her vagina and lodge itself in her bloodstream, potentially blocking a blood vessel. This very un-cool maneuver can be fatal, so keep that one out of your repertoire.

Also, never be rough on a woman's vaginal area. As I've said before, a woman's vaginal area, much like a man's penis, is very sensitive. Be gentle when kissing, licking, and sucking, and don't bite on anything unless specifically instructed. Here, apparently, is another move that women consider very un-cool, according to my friend Brooke:

> "Hold on. John, since I know this
> discussion is going to wind up in a future

book, can you please also put this in your book? Tell guys that it's very difficult for a woman to cum through sex. And that if a guy wants to be invited back in my bedroom in the future, he better make me cum.

I don't have a problem with sex; I actually enjoy sex a lot. But I don't routinely cum from sex. Most guys are usually done in a few minutes, and then they roll over and go to sleep. I've only met one guy, Rick, who actually knew what to do.

After he had cum, knowing that I still hadn't, Rick went down on me. It was SO intense. I was already very turned on, so it only took Rick about a minute and a half. He ran his tongue all over me until I was orgasming in sheer ecstasy.

Now Rick has a season's pass to my bedroom. He's welcome whenever he wants! Why can't more guys be like that?!"

You should have heard the room erupt with laughter at Brooke's 'season's pass' comment! While my female friends certainly seem to be big fans of oral sex, guys often tell me:

"The girl I'm dating refuses to let me give her oral sex. We've slept together and done everything else, but she won't let me perform oral sex on her. It's like she's denying herself this intense pleasure. Why is this?"

For all of you guys who have found yourself in this seemingly peculiar predicament, you're not alone. I've actually found that there are quite a few women out there who have inhibitions about oral sex and do not want a guy performing oral sex on them. Unfortunately, this is often preventing her from having an orgasm at all. Here are some basic guidelines if your girlfriend or wife refuses oral sex:

First, only attempt to perform oral sex on her in a room that is pitch black with darkness. Many women are insecure about their bodies and don't like the fact that you're looking up at them and can see their entire body when you're performing oral sex on them. A good first step is attempting oral sex only in a dark room in which the woman knows that you can't see her.

A woman might refuse oral sex simply because she has received such bad attempts at oral sex in the past since, unfortunately, most guys exert so little effort and consequently just aren't that good at performing oral sex. She may have experienced guys who put too much pressure on her clitoris and ended up hurting her. In this case, it is up to you to show her that oral sex leads to tremendous pleasure by performing it correctly.

Additionally, a lot of women have heard that the vaginal area smells bad and that vaginal fluids are very unpleasant. Many women are simply embarrassed that they smell or taste bad and thus don't want anyone going down there. It is very important to keep in mind a woman's need for reassurance at this point. As you perform oral sex on a woman, tell her how great she tastes. A simple one line compliment such as, "Honey, you taste so good," can provide the reassurance that a woman needs in order for her to permit you to perform oral sex on her.

Another good tip is get the woman as highly aroused as possible, through kissing, licking, and stroking her lips, face, neck, shoulders, breasts, nipples, arms, fingers, stomach, thighs, and calves. Then move on and insert a finger or two into her vagina and lightly massage her clitoris with your thumb. Try to massage her G-spot if you can find it. Keep doing this until she is sufficiently aroused, possibly even on the verge of orgasm. But do not let her orgasm (yet). It is in this highly aroused state that a woman will be most likely to try something new.

While continuing to use your fingers and maintaining this high state of arousal, slowly go down and kiss her stomach, belly button, and work your way down to her thighs. While you're down there, flick at her clitoris a time or two with your tongue. More than likely, the extreme sensation she'll feel when you flick at her clitoris will help overcome her previous inhibitions about receiving oral sex. Continue on and bring her to orgasm with your tongue using the procedures outlined above. Once she has experienced that tremendous clitoral orgasm for the first time, I doubt that she will continue to reject oral sex in the future. In fact, after experiencing an orgasm in this manner for the first time, she will probably beg you for more.

Now that you're an expert at performing oral sex, you still have to deal with the fact that your woman probably doesn't meet your expectations when it comes to performing oral sex on you. We at The Nice Guys' Institute™ are currently working on a report on the very delicate topic of instructing your woman how to improve her oral sex technique. When we're finished, we'll post our report on www.TheNiceGuysGuide.com, or include it in a sequel.

Visit the site often as we are constantly updating it with new content, including downloadable e-books and e-reports, audio tapes and CDs, and video cassettes and DVDs packed with our latest discoveries. We also maintain information on our web site about upcoming coaching sessions, course offerings, and speaking engagements. Additionally, we encourage readers to e-mail us, either through our web site, or at TheNiceGuys@TheNiceGuysGuide.com. Finally, please also come by and sign up for our free newsletter to receive the hottest tips to help nice guys like you make themselves more attractive to women WITHOUT turning into jerks!

Chapter 8 – The Nice Guys' Guide™ to Getting Your Ex Back

One of the most common e-mails we receive at *The Nice Guys' Institute*™ always seems to follow the same pattern:

> "My girlfriend and I broke up two months ago. It was kind of her decision. We still talk a lot, but she says we should see other people. I want to be with her, not with other people. I've told her this, too. What should I do? I feel like if I date other girls, it will end up pushing her away, and I don't want to do that."

For all you guys out there in search of the answer to this question, my best advice is to see the movie *Swingers*. What a great movie. The premise of the movie is that, as a guy, the way to get your ex-girlfriend back is to get over her. That your ex-girlfriend will come running back to you the moment you are actually over her - not the moment you pretend to be over her, not the moment you tell yourself you're over her, but the moment you really are over her.

When is this moment? This is the moment at which you really no longer care that your ex-girlfriend wants you back. It is the point in time when you go through the day and no longer think about your ex-girlfriend. It's the moment when her birthday approaches, and you don't even remember it (though I suppose a lot of guys do that anyway – who knows, that might even explain why she became your *ex*-girlfriend!). It's the moment when you go out at night and don't even wonder what she's doing tonight. It's the moment when you can go out with another girl without thinking about your ex-girlfriend. This is the moment when your ex-girlfriend will want you back.

Here's what we've learned (and women, listen up – this applies to both sexes): The number one way to get an ex back is to move on with your life. Nothing is more unattractive to either sex than an ex constantly calling, apologizing for things, wanting to work things out, and begging for you to come back. The way that the human psyche works makes that extremely unattractive.

On the flip side, what is extremely attractive is the realization that your ex-boyfriend or ex-girlfriend no longer needs you. Guys: When a woman sees that you've stopped calling and e-mailing her and realizes that you're probably dating another woman, that's when she starts to become attracted to you again. That's when she starts thinking about you and realizes how much she misses you.

For those of you whose heart has been broken and are struggling a little bit right now, my best advice to you is to move on and genuinely look to date other people. One of two things will happen: Either you'll find someone else who you get along with better than your ex, or your ex will want you back. Who knows, if you're lucky, it's possible that both will happen, making you the envy of many other men.

My good friend Diana had this to say about her ex-boyfriend:

> "I originally broke up with Joseph because he was starting to get too clingy. I just needed some space. When I first broke up with him, he was a mess. I did it in the nicest way possible. I told him, 'Hey, I love you, but I need some time apart. I need to think things over. I need to realize what I'm looking for in life. I need some space.' And oh, did that crush him.
>
> He would go out, get trashed, and drunk-dial me. He would call and e-mail me to see how I was doing. He was truly pathetic and annoying during that first month after our break-up. I even ran into him once at a bar, and he just started yelling at me, telling me how awful I was and how I had ruined his life. Let me tell you . . . that was really attractive.
>
> At that point, I had moved on and was dating someone else, Jim. Things were going OK. Jim and I had been dating for a few weeks when suddenly I realized I hadn't heard from Joseph in over a month. I hadn't seen him. I hadn't heard from him. All I knew was that he had just started dating someone else, according to a friend of mine.
>
> I don't know what happened, but the more I went out with Jim, the more I started to realize how much I missed Joseph and how Joseph was the guy I wanted to be with. I really don't know what it was; I guess it was just that over time, as I spent more time apart from Joseph and started

dating another guy, I realized how much I missed him. So I e-mailed him to see how he was doing. Things progressed slowly, but we eventually ended up getting back together. And we're still together today!"

The moral to the story? Keep living your life when your heart gets broken. Things will get better. They might even be better than they ever were before – maybe even with the same woman!

AFTERWORD

Becoming a Nice Guy™ is incredible! When you approach women by showing genuine, sincere interest in them, rather than bragging about yourself, women will really enjoy being around you. When you have patience, instead of being the aggressive male that so many guys are, women will be amazed and shocked. When you invite women to do fun things that you know interest them, they will gladly want to go out with you. When you focus your dates on having a fun time, and making great conversation, rather than trying to impress women with how much money you can spend on them, your dates will be intrigued that you're so much different from other guys they've dated. Women will *want* to date you, *want* to sleep with you, and *want* to enter into relationships with you. It will change your life, as it has changed ours.

The next step is up to you. Being a Nice Guy is extremely powerful, so don't waste any more time. Try it today – at a bar, at a party, in a bookstore, wherever – the possibilities are endless! Refer back to *The Nice Guys' Guide*™ when you have questions, or shoot us an e-mail at TheNiceGuys@TheNiceGuysGuide.com. Tell us your stories. Tell us all about the great girl you met by using the techniques in this book and how she *gave* you her contact info without you even asking. We'll put the best stories on our website!

We wish *you* as much success being a Nice Guy, as we have experienced ourselves.

Good luck,

The Nice Guy™ & The Nice Guys™

Glossary

Bothersome Environments – One of three types of
environments in which to meet women (the other
two are Naturally-Inviting Environments and
Moderately-Inviting Environments). Bothersome
environments are the toughest environments in
which to meet women, because you are
interrupting them from some other activity.
Unfortunately, bothersome environments are
also the most common places to meet women.
These include: bars, bookstores, concerts,
subways, buses, restaurants, coffee shops,
grocery stores, festivals, parks, and walking
down the street.

CCR – It is the premise of *Make Every Girl Want You*™.
It is an acronym that stands for Compliments,
Compassion, and Reassurance. By sincerely
complimenting women, showing them
compassion, and reassuring them that things
will be ok in times of need, you make women feel
good about themselves. This makes women want

to be around you. When combined with a positive, confident attitude, women will *WANT* you.

Category 1 Guy – One of the three categories of guys who traditionally got women. Category 1 guys are really good-looking.

Category 2 Guy – One of the three categories of guys who traditionally got women. Category 2 guys are rich.

Category 3 Guy – One of the three categories of guys who traditionally got women. Category 3 guys are famous (including local celebrities).

Category 4 Guy – The new category of guys who get women: a Nice Guy.

Direct Vouch – A positive statement about you from a female friend of yours to a female friend of hers. An example is, "Jen, you have to meet my friend Dave!! He is really awesome!!" Receiving *direct vouches* is one of the best ways to befriend new women quickly. As you develop into a true Nice Guy, you will receive more and more of these.

Dudefest – You know what this is! It's when you end up at a party or event with mostly guys and few single women. True Nice Guys know how to handle this annoying situation properly.

Emotion Matching – This is the key to compassion. By matching a woman's mood, whether it is happy or sad, she feels connected to you emotionally.

Golden Rule of CCR – If you don't have anything CCR to say, don't say anything at all!

Indirect Vouch – This vouch occurs when you and the girl you've just met have a close mutual female friend. This girl that you've just met will be much more receptive toward you knowing that you are good friends with a friend of hers.

Man of CCR – This is what you become once you've read and implemented what we suggest in *Make Every Girl Want You*™. This man compliments women, shows compassion toward them, and reassures them. He projects a positive, confident attitude toward women. As a result, women love this type of guy. This, in turn, makes even more women want him. Women want a Man of CCR as much as one who is rich, famous, or really good-looking!

Moderately-Inviting Environments – One of three types of environments in which to meet women (the other two are Naturally-Inviting Environments and Bothersome Environments). Moderately-inviting environments are, as the name might suggest, moderately easy places to meet women. Some examples include: a co-ed sports team, a wine-tasting class, the local chapter of your alumni association, and a church or temple. When women are in these environments, their primary purpose often isn't to meet new people. They are usually, however, aware that they will meet new people through these groups and clubs, and thus are moderately inviting toward men who may approach them.

Naturally-Inviting Environments – One of three types of environments in which to meet women (the other two are Moderately-Inviting Environments and Bothersome Environments). Naturally-Inviting environments are the easiest environments in which to meet women, such as at a party where a mutual friend is likely to introduce you.

Relinquishing Short-Term Sexual Desire – Conveying an attitude toward women that you are interested in them as a person, *not* as a sex object.

Subconscious Vouch – This subtle vouch is extremely powerful. This vouch occurs when you bring a fun, attractive female friend to an event with you, and other women there see you with her. Subconsciously these other women think you get along well with all women. They will naturally desire you more because they see other fun, attractive women who also enjoy your company.

Third-Party Compliment – A compliment you say to one person regarding someone who is not present. It is the complete opposite of talking badly behind someone's back. It is such a great feeling the first time a female says, "You know, you never have a bad thing to say about anyone. I love the fact that you are always so positive. It's truly refreshing to be around someone who always sees the good in people."

Vouch – The positive response a female has toward you as a result of something positive she has seen or heard about you from other females. There are three types of vouches—the direct vouch, the indirect vouch, and the subconscious vouch.

Appendix A – Questions to Ask a Woman That You Have Just Met

Here are some topics for discussion as you're getting to know a girl. These will allow you to make great conversation, and provide you with ideas for things to invite her to. Do not *ever* ask these questions rapid-fire. These are simply meant to spark conversation, not to be asked sequentially. Inevitably, a question will send the two of you off on some random tangent, allowing you to learn exciting things about her that you never would have thought to ask. That is exactly the purpose of these questions. If you find yourself going through this list in order, then this girl probably doesn't want to talk to you right now. Go talk to someone else.

Background
- So are you from <this city>?
- Oh, where are you originally from?

- Do you like <city you're from>?
- Have you lived there your whole life?
- Where else have you lived?

Current City

- So why'd you come to <this city>?
- How long have you lived here?
- What part of town do you live in?
- What part of town do you normally go out in?
- How often do you go out? (Politely)

Career / Job

- So where do you work?
- Do you like it?
- How long have you worked there?
- Where did you work before that?

School

- So did you go to school around here?
- Where did you go to school?
- Why did you choose <school>?
- Did you like it?
- What did you major in?
- Why did you choose <major>?
- Did you like it?
- Have you thought about going back to school?
- To study what?
- Where have you thought about applying?

Friends

- So, do you have a lot of friends from school who live here in <city>?

- Where did most of your friends end up moving?
  - (Try to lead into discussion of cities you've visited or where your friends live)

Family

- So does your family live in <city>?
- Do you visit them often?
- Do you have any siblings?
- Younger or older?
- Where do they live?
- Are you close to them?
  - (Discuss your own siblings, their ages, where they live, and how close you are)

Travel

- Ask if she's been to any cool nearby places, such as a nearby beach, ski resort, National Park, campground, city, tourist attraction, college, vineyard, or lake. Try to get a feel for what she enjoys doing and where she hasn't yet been but would love to go.

Sports

- So did you go to football/basketball games at <school>?
- Are you a sports fan?
- What sports do you follow (if any)?
- Do you play any sports?

Entertainment

- What's your favorite TV show?
- What TV shows do you watch regularly?

- Have you seen any good movies lately?
- What are your favorite types of movies?
- What is your all-time favorite movie?
- Are there any movies out now that you want to see? (Try to be subtle; don't imply too much)

Appendix B – Date Ideas

Here are some ideas for dates, or just fun things to do with a group of mixed-sex friends.

Nature
- Boating
- Fishing
- Canoeing
- Lake
- Hiking
- Camping
- Scenic drive
- Beach
- Skiing / snow boarding
- Tubing
- Caverns
- Jet ski
- Water ski
- Biking

- Picnic
- Roller-blading / Roller-skating
- Walk a girl's dog in a park
- Fly a kite in a park
- Paddle boating
- Barbecue at a friend's pool (or apartment complex's pool)
- Botanical Garden
- Park or other nice outdoor spot
- Walk around nearby college campus
- Apple picking

Culture

- Museum
- Aquarium
- Zoo
- Vineyard
- Play / musical
- Other cultural spots (check local guidebooks)

Amusement / Entertainment

- Theme park
- Movie theater
- Rent a movie
- Miniature golf
- Bowling
- Shoot pool
- Comedy club
- Ice skating
- Water park
- Concert
- Drive-in movie
- Karaoke
- Murder mystery dinner
- Watch horse racing

- Watch polo match

Play sports

- Volleyball
- Tennis (become doubles partners)
- Driving range
- Batting cage
- Racquetball

Sporting Events

- Pro, college, or minor league

Seasonal

- Outdoor concerts in the summertime
- Horse races in the spring/summer
- Halloween
  - Hayride
  - Pumpkin picking
- Christmas
  - Watch the Nutcracker
  - See Christmas lights

Food / Drinks

- Grab lunch during the week
- Sunday brunch
- Grab a drink after work
- Ice cream
- Sushi
- Pastry shop
- Coffee shop
- Grab dessert
- Cook for a girl (***Girls love this!)

- Cook with a girl, or ask her to show you how to make a recipe. (You should at least be minimally capable in the kitchen to request this)
- Order Chinese food or a pizza

Shopping

- Local mall
- Popular shopping district (may be out of town)

Appendix C – Recurring Event Ideas

Softball

Here are some guidelines for building a softball team:

- Join a local city or county league; it should be quite inexpensive.
- Make sure you enter a co-ed, non-competitive league. Do not make the mistake of entering a competitive league. This will scare off and annoy the girls.
- You may have a choice of season length; try to keep the season to about 2 months. Games will probably be weekly.
- Roster size is usually 20-25 people; 10 players usually play at once.

- Invite 7 or 8 guys to join the team; save the rest of the roster spots for girls. Try not to invite any highly competitive guys. This will really annoy the women.
- Go to the batting cage as a team or call a team practice before the season; this will be a good excuse to get all of the girls together.
- Send out a weekly e-mail the day of a game, reminding everyone of the game time, location, and directions. Ask people to respond if they will attend. Include your cell phone number in the e-mail; inevitably someone will get lost or forget the directions.
- You won't have a problem getting guys to attend; if you ever fall short, you can easily find a male friend to play for the day (guys love softball and guys love women—what guy wouldn't join in?)
- You will have problems getting girls to attend. You will probably need to call around each week just to convince 5 girls to show up.
- This used to frustrate us, until we started using it to our benefit. We would purposely try to fall a girl or two short each week so that we could invite a girl we'd recently met to play for the day.
- Do *not* take winning seriously. It is quite possible that you will be really bad. The girls don't mind losing. What girls do mind are highly competitive guys. Don't be that guy. Once again, try not to invite any highly competitive guys to play.
- Consider drinking during the games. This probably won't be permitted, since you'll be playing in a city/county park or on school grounds. Mix something up in a cooler and sneak it in. If anyone asks, just say it's juice.
- The best drink is something sweet with a lot of sugar. We recommend mixing 1-½ gallons of fruit punch with a handle of vodka and a 7-lb. bag of ice. Beer or non-sweet mixed drinks will dehydrate everyone.

- Don't forget to bring the equipment (bats and balls) to each game, or appoint someone to be responsible for it. If you're drinking, bring 25 paper or plastic cups each week.
- Appoint someone on the team to coach. Choose someone who knows softball well, but isn't highly competitive. This will relieve you of the responsibility of keeping track of who hasn't played yet, and listening to people (girls) whine about what position you've stuck them in.
- Have fun with it! It's a bit of work, but in the end it's a lot of fun and of great benefit to you!

Wine-tasting

Here are some guidelines for organizing wine tastings:

- Gather a small group of friends (maybe 10 people) who all know each other.
- Get together once a week or once every other week.
- Taste a new type of wine each week. (Some popular reds are Cabernet Sauvignon, Merlot, Shiraz, Pinot Noir, and Chianti; some popular whites are Chardonnay, Sauvignon Blanc, Pinot Grigio, and Riesling)
- Have a different person host it each week; rotate through the group so that everyone hosts once.
- Each week, have everyone bring a bottle of the chosen grape. It's actually better to state that there should be 1 bottle for every 2 people (any more than this is too much wine). Don't state 1 bottle per couple; this will dissuade single girls from attending.
- With the "1 bottle for every 2 people" rule in place, this makes it easy to call up a girl you've recently met and ask if she'd like to join you for the evening. Tell her you'll get the wine. If things go well, you can suggest that she get the wine next week.

- As people arrive, have the host put each bottle in a brown bag. Write a number on the outside of each bag. Give everyone a wine glass and have everyone rate each wine by number. At the end, remove the brown bags and let people see which wines they liked best. Then let your friends drink from whichever bottle they please the rest of the evening.
- The host may wish to request that people bring their own wine glasses.
- It is a nice touch for the host to serve appetizers. Cheese and crackers are always popular with wine.
- Send out a weekly e-mail reminding everyone of the host, location, directions, grape, and time. Build enthusiasm by stating how much fun it will be!
- Run the wine-tasting events for 10-12 weeks, and then move on to another activity.
- Wine tasting is a lot of fun. The group size will probably grow each week.

Activity Night

A varying-activity night, in which you get together the same night every week but for a different activity, is also a lot of fun. Here are some good activities to try:

- Ice skating
- Night skiing
- Movie rental
- Bowling
- Potluck dinner
- Pool tournament
- Bar night
- Board/card game
- Miniature golf
- Wine and cheesecake night

Other Recurring Events

Here are some more ideas for recurring events. If you come up with any more, please e-mail us and let us know:

- Get everyone to take a weekly cooking class together
- Get everyone to take a weekly dancing class together (girls love this)
- Have a monthly potluck dinner; host every month or rotate hosts
- Movie night
- Have everyone gather one night a week to watch the popular TV shows
- Plan around actual events, such as a weekly concert series

Quick Order Form

Web Orders: www.TheNiceGuysGuide.com
E-mail Orders: sales@TheNiceGuysGuide.com
Fax Orders: see www.TheNiceGuysGuide.com
Telephone Orders: see www.TheNiceGuysGuide.com
Mail Orders: see www.TheNiceGuysGuide.com

Name: _____

Address: _____

City: _____ State: _____ Zip: _____

Telephone: _____

E-mail Address: _____

Shipping & Handling: $2.95/book for all orders in U.S. (total is $17.90/book in U.S., except in Virginia)

Sales tax: Please add 4.5% for products shipped to Virginia (total is $18.57/book in Virginia)

Quantity: _____ **Total: $**_____
I understand that I may return any products for a full refund—for any reason, no questions asked.

Payment: ____check ____ credit card:
Payment must accompany orders. Allow 3 weeks for delivery.

____Visa ____MasterCard

Card number: _____

Name on card: _____Exp. Date: _____

Signature: _____